...e...'s Method

Tyson Fury is the undefeated lineal heavyweight champion of the world. Born and raised in Manchester, Fury weighed just 1lb at birth after being born three months premature. His father John named him after Mike Tyson.

From Irish traveller heritage, the 'Gypsy King' is undefeated in 28 professional fights, winning 27 with 19 knockouts, and drawing once. In 2015, he famously stunned long-time champion Wladimir Klitschko to win the WBA, IBF and WBO world heavyweight titles. But he was forced to vacate the belts because of issues with drugs, alcohol and mental health, and did not fight again for more than two years. Most thought he was done with boxing forever. Until an amazing comeback fight with Deontay Wilder in December 2018. It was an instant classic, ending in a split-decision tie. Tyson was victorious in the second fight against Deontay Wilder in February 2020, defeating his opponent by seventh-round technical knockout. In October 2021, Tyson concluded the trilogy with victory against Deontay Wilder by an emphatic eleventh-round technical knockout.

Outside of the ring, Tyson Fury is a mental health ambassador

TYSON FURY

The Furious Method

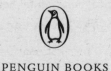

PENGUIN BOOKS

PENGUIN BOOKS

UK | USA | Canada | Ireland | Australia
India | New Zealand | South Africa

Penguin Books is part of the Penguin Random House group of companies
whose addresses can be found at global.penguinrandomhouse.com

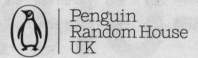

Penguin
Random House
UK

First published by Century 2020
Published in Penguin Books 2021

001

Typeset by Jouve (UK), Milton Keynes
Printed and bound in Great Britain by Clays Ltd, Elcograf S.p.A.

The authorised representative in the EEA is Penguin Random House Ireland,
Morrison Chambers, 32 Nassau Street, Dublin D02 YH68

A CIP catalogue record for this book is available from the British Library

ISBN: 978-1-529-15634-8

I had to get back up.
I had to show the world that nothing is impossible.
For all the people who suffer with mental health problems,
I dedicate this book to you. If I can come back from the
brink, you can too. So get back up! Seek professional help.
And let's do this together, as a team.

CONTENTS

PROLOGUE

22 February 2020: MGM Grand Garden Arena, Las Vegas, USA

It's showtime. Nearly midnight in Vegas. My second fight against the big dosser Deontay Wilder, the biggest knockout merchant in boxing history. This is the most hotly anticipated bout here since Lennox Lewis faced Evander Holyfield twenty years ago. Outside it's a cool evening; inside the arena it's a cauldron of expectation. They've had to lock the doors at the MGM Grand Garden to keep people out. A capacity audience of 17,000 people is buzzing, the darkness popping with the flashes of camera phones. At ringside there are celebrities including Michael J. Fox, Magic Johnson, Triple H from the WWE, and the chef Gordon Ramsay – the latter two kindly wish me well before the fight. Punters are paying up to £13,000 for a front-row ticket. My fans are singing 'You big dosser!' against the Wilder crowd shouting 'Bomb squad!' I feed off their energy.

I always enjoy coming up with ideas for my ring walks; they're like my miniature productions. I pick songs and outfits that mean something to me and that people can relate to. My first fight in Las Vegas in 2019 I came out in the stars and stripes outfit Apollo Creed wore in *Rocky IV*, with James Brown singing 'Living in America'. For my next fight I was boxing on Mexican Independence Day, so I wore a sombrero and had a mariachi band. For tonight's battle I'm dressed as a king in a crown and cape, sitting on a golden throne and carried into the arena. I'm accompanied by the syrupy voice of Patsy Cline singing 'Crazy' – an ironic nod to my mental health battles!

I'm enjoying every second of the build-up to Fury vs Wilder 2. This is my moment, my chance to be a showman on the world's biggest stage. The Gypsy King never disappoints. There are no butterflies in my stomach, I have nothing to fear. Mentally, I've already won this fight, which is most of the battle. I'm ready for a twelve-round war or a one-round knockout. It's my time to shine.

It's been fourteen months since me and the Bronze Bomber last 'danced', which was a controversial draw even though anyone who watched it knows I was the winner. Tonight's fight will be a very different story. I know what needs to be done and, like Muhammad Ali, I've made no bones about telling Wilder that I'm going for a KO in two rounds. At last night's weigh-in I clocked in at 19 stone 7 pounds (273 pounds), Wilder at 16 stone 7 pounds (231 pounds), so I have a good forty pounds on him. He's the heaviest weight he's been in years; maybe he's looking for more strength in our clinches, throwing shots on the inside. Both of us are heavier than we were last time, but there's more to this game than weight. I'm the master of mind games and I've already burrowed deep into his head. At our last press conference a few days ago, I told Wilder: 'You're terrified. Your little knees are knocking. Keep that belt warm for me!' The upshot was that we ended up shoving one another about the stage. So, come the weigh-in, Bob Arum, my promoter, and the Nevada Commission wisely made the decision to keep us far apart.

There are two things that can happen when a shaken champion like Wilder takes a rematch with a fighter who has schooled him in the ring. Either he does something drastically different in style to redeem himself, or he sticks with the routine that didn't work for him last time and walks straight back into the same nightmare. For this fight, I hear Wilder's camp have been working on his precision; he's going need it if he wants to get close to this slippery 6 foot 9 eel. Fourteen months ago, I gave the Bronze Bomber his first taste of trouble with the draw in LA, upsetting the symmetry of his perfect record: thirty-nine wins by way of knockout, no losses, with nineteen of his victims impressively dispatched within the first round. Since then he's added another two knockouts to his record, another one of which was in the first round. But I'm the one with the mental edge here, the boxing

IQ, the hand speed and fancy footwork. Wilder can't cope with my personality or my fighting skills.

It feels like a million thoughts pass through my head, but I think of the heritage of my fighting family and it calms me; warriors past and present willing me on to make history tonight. You see, I come from fighting royalty and there are Gypsy Kings – meaning the best bareknuckle fighter of the Gypsies – on both sides of my family. On my dad's side, Bartley Gorman was the last in a long line of Gorman Gypsy Kings. For twenty years he ruled supreme – from 1972 to 1992 – and would take on brawls from all challengers. As a ten-year-old, my dad witnessed him at the Doncaster Races facing up to a mob of thirty men with iron bars, hammers and knives; he'd gone there to fight one man, but was ambushed by a gang. One man against thirty. But he didn't cave in, he just kept going, dropping them like flies even as they cut him to ribbons. He had the option to walk away but instead he said grimly to himself, 'this is my moment of truth.'

Now this is my moment against Wilder. It feels weird not having my former trainer Ben Davison with me, as we'd become an inseparable team. I wouldn't be here without him, as he helped me so much during my comeback from the depths of depression. We're still the best of mates, but for certain fights you need different styles and what I did before against Wilder back in late

4

November 2018 clearly wasn't enough to win conclusively (though most scorecards had me ahead). To nail this fight and finish it the way I want to — up close and toe-to-toe — I've had to channel something else: aggression. And nobody does controlled aggression like the legendary Kronk Gym in Detroit. The battered heavy bags I've destroyed and knocked off their hooks are evidence of the explosive style I've been developing. Let's see if the dosser still calls me 'pillow fists' at the end of this fight!

I'm nearly at the ring now. I'm up off my gold throne, on my feet and blowing gloved kisses to the crowd as 'Crazy' plays a second time. I can almost taste battle now, like when you smell a storm coming. Our procession finally stops, and I slowly descend the steps as calmly as if I was on my way to sit down at the table for a Sunday roast. The crowd roars as I walk to the ring and climb over the ropes. Vegas: once the working home of Elvis Presley, Tom Jones and Frank Sinatra, and now my home fighting turf. I feel loved by the Yanks; they've taken me in to their hearts. They seem to welcome comeback artists, and also seem to like that I look and talk like a normal bloke.

From a cloud of dry ice and beams of purple light emerges Wilder, also wearing a crown, and decked out in glittering black armour. True to form, he's hiding behind another mask as he does for all his entrances, this one with glowing red eyes. Somewhere between a *Lord of the Rings* villain and the rabbit from *Donnie Darko*, he looks extraordinarily . . . daft. Slowly, those red eyes get closer, but they don't unsettle me. The WBC reigning champion raises his gloved fists to the heavens as if he is charging them with lightning, and he climbs in to join me for *unfinished business* . . .

Wilder seems stiff, even tense behind the mask. Andy Lee, my cousin and number two coach, was in his dressing room earlier to check that his wraps were correctly applied. This is to ensure no hardening materials are present in the gauze padding around the knuckle area (including sulphur and calcium, two of the ingredients in plaster of Paris). Andy said it was tense and quiet in there, as opposed to the positive vibes in my room. Apparently, you could have cut the atmosphere with a knife.

As Jimmy Lennon announces the fight in his rich baritone, I'm throwing shapes and savouring the moment like a glass of chilled champagne, loving every second of every minute. Then the bell goes for the promoters, cut men and coaches to exit the ring – that lonely, desolate fighter's square which I've known most of my life. In a little over half an hour's time – or if my plan goes the way it should, much less – the blue canvas will be scattered with pools of blood, hopefully not mine. I see my wife, Paris, at ringside, dazzling in a ruby dress. I exchange a glance with 'SugarHill' Steward, my head coach from the Kronk Gym. Ali once said: 'The fight is won or lost far away from witnesses – behind the lines, in the gym, and out there on the road, long before I dance under those lights.' And SugarHill knows just as I know that we've done the work we need to; now it's time for me to enjoy myself. Train hard, fight easy.

Earlier that day, seven of us had gathered in the lounge of the house we were staying at in Vegas as SugarHill went over the fight plan. It wasn't complicated. I'm to hold the centre of the ring, stalk Wilder relentlessly so he's always on the back foot, while throwing rounds of heavy punches at him. It'll be pure educated aggression. I can't let him come forward and build any momentum, allowing him to be at his most dangerous. If you're wondering if I lost any sleep the night before the fight trying to second-guess what Wilder might come up with this time to silence me, all I can say is I slept like a baby. Nuff said. It doesn't interest me what someone else is planning to do to me; let them plan all they like. As Mike Tyson once said, and tonight I can see him sitting ringside in my corner as a show of support: 'Everyone has a plan until they get punched in the face.'

Back in the ring. Moments before the bell. Kenny Bayless, the referee, calls us fighters together before seconds out, and as Wilder presents his gloves to touch mine, I make him wait a beat before I bring mine up. Up close, I can see his tattoos of rosaries, psalms, crosses and Chinese lettering. Now his eyes are fixed on mine. *Just another bum with a pair of gloves on*, I think to myself. *Time to go to work!*

As the bell for Round One rings, I sprint out to the middle of the ring to control the action, working the feint and hitting the Bronze Bomber with solid spearing jabs. I've been telling him throughout the build-up to the fight that I'm going to be dropping my own bombs. Maybe he didn't believe me, but now that it's happening, Wilder seems surprised by the weight and power of my shots. I'm moving him back, scoring him with jabs and as I get right into his face there's a look of panic in the whites of his eyes. He's not used to being backed up like this; he can't punch off his back foot. It's out of his comfort zone and beyond his skillset.

I have the greatest of respect for Wilder, this man who I've verbally danced with, mocked and faced-off with over the last week. That's all part of the theatre and brings a bit of drama into people's lives. It's more thrilling if everyone thinks we're arch enemies and that we hate each other. But there's no hate from me. You have to admire a man who only started boxing eleven years ago at the age of nineteen, with the sole purpose of making enough money to take care of his baby girl, who has spina bifida. We are so blessed to have the NHS taking care of us in the UK; if you can't afford medical insurance in the US, you're screwed.

I witnessed that first hand with the many ill and homeless people on Skid Row in LA in the lead-up to the first Wilder fight; it bummed the hell out of me. Like those people, I know what it's like to be a vulnerable person. Although I wasn't without a roof over my head, during my depression I'd had the same drug and alcohol problems that many of these people who had landed on the street had experienced. Just because someone is ill or addicted it doesn't make them a loser and they shouldn't be forgotten. People need help. I had help and lots of it; I wouldn't be here without it. I respect Wilder for helping his daughter and for inspiring others to get help, too.

I also respect Wilder's grit. When he was trying to make it as a pro, he worked himself beyond exhaustion driving a Budweiser delivery truck, some days for seventeen hours. During this time, he slept in his car outside the gym, training at every spare moment. He was in a hurry to learn his craft, his motivation was strong: his little girl's illness worsening. Within a year and a half of putting on his first boxing glove, Wilder was invited to the Olympics and won a bronze medal. It's amazing what you can achieve when you are focused and when time is against you – a lesson for all of us.

And I'll tell you one final thing about Wilder. Years ago, back in Detroit when I was being trained by Manny Steward, the wise old trainer predicted that one day two young punks would dominate the heavyweight division. The first one was Tyson Fury. The second one? The man with the freakish strength and the devastating right hand that feels like a sock full of snooker balls whacking you on the temple: Deontay Wilder, of course. Wilder's punches hurt more than they should do. How else can a man weighing an average of 210 pounds regularly drop guys of 260 pounds or more? Apparently his grandma once said he was anointed and special. I don't know about anointed, but he's definitely special.

Back to the fight, and for all my respect for my opponent, I'm still going to put Wilder's arse down and knock his lights out. Throughout the opening two rounds, I'm dominating using my orthodox left foot forward as a range measurer. Wilder doesn't know if it's a feint jab, a one-two or a straight right hand coming next. I pressure him, not permitting him a second to compose himself or come up with a plan. Not that he ever seems to have one. There's arrogance for you. That's the problem with knockout merchants: they're so spoilt by getting their own way in the first few rounds, they never prepare for the long haul and the box of skills they'll need to employ over twelve rounds. The best way to beat a bully is to take the fight right to them, bully the bully, and that is exactly what I'm doing. In the last thirty seconds of the second round, Wilder attempts to land an overhead bomb and misses by an Alabama mile. So much for the precision training his camp were supposed to have been working on.

Towards the end of the third round, I hit Wilder with a quicksilver left-right hook combo, and literally whip him onto the canvas. The crowd are up on their feet cheering, scenting blood and victory, like the crowds in Rome thousands of years ago who paid to watch gladiators cut one another to pieces.

Wilder springs up off the floor like the warrior he is.

What were you saying about my pillow fists, Deontay?

I trot to the corner and wait while the ref gives Wilder the count. I feel sprightly and light on my feet. Adrenaline is coursing through my veins; it's hard to describe the euphoria. I haven't felt this good in years. Standing in the ring right now, everything in my life feels on track. All of the pain, the suffering and the dedication during my comeback was worth it. My family and friends are all watching – in the arena or back at home. I feel them with me. I'm thankful for everyone who got me back here.

I'm not here now to humiliate Wilder, nor do I want to slowly turn the screw and play this torture out over twelve rounds. Ali once said in an interview that he was a sportsman and that he took no pleasure in drawing blood or making another man suffer – the sweet science of boxing isn't about that. I agree with him, I just want to finish this quickly. There are still thirty seconds left in the round as the ref waves Wilder back into the contest. A lot can happen in thirty seconds. I feel great, but it only takes one punch . . .

INTRODUCTION

I was 50 per cent of myself the first time I fought Deontay Wilder. But when I faced the Bronze Bomber for the second time, in February 2020, and beat him, shocking the world, I can honestly say I have never been more perfectly prepared and well-conditioned for a fight. Everything worked smoothly in the run-up to that night: my training camp, sparring partners, diet and mindset. I was 100 per cent firing on all cylinders.

In this book I want to share with you the secrets and methods I employed both in my comeback against Wilder, and my comeback in life. I'll show you how I was able to create positive personal change and how you can go about doing the same.

For me, there's no sensation in the world that can match the feeling of going into battle with another high-performance athlete at world-class level. It feels amazing because I know I've done all the work, I'm where I'm supposed to be, and it's all down to me to make history. Are they going to write 'Tyson Fury lost by knockout' or 'Tyson Fury won'?

I appreciate not everyone will share the same desire to get into the ring and knock ten bells out of someone. But I believe the building blocks of my successful comeback over depression and weight issues to become heavyweight champion of the world once again can be useful for anyone. Remember, I look like an average Joe: bald and a bit fat around the midriff. In the depths of my depression I was suicidal and weighed 28 stone. But thanks to the support from my family and friends, and by seeking professional help and focusing on a positive outlook on life, I got healthy in body and mind. I hope you haven't been through what I have, but I do hope the challenges I have overcome will resonate with challenges that you have faced, or are facing. I'll draw on my experiences from boxing but also from out of the ring. Far from being exclusive to 6 foot 9 giants, these simple approaches and life tips are there for all of us to access.

Over the course of twelve chapters and twelve rounds, we'll address being knocked down and how to get back up again with resilience (all the wiser and stronger for it). We'll look at the transformative power of exercise, and how to find your natural fighting (and living) weight, with tips to help you stay happy and to keep the weight off in the future. Together, we'll re-train our minds to create a positive mindset. Along the way we'll challenge ourselves with goal-setting, we'll tackle self-doubt and we'll learn to fully believe in ourselves. At the start of each chapter, I've also included a cardio workout for you to try each morning, based on similar workouts that I like to do.

What made me sit down and write this book? In March 2020, the global pandemic turned our lives into a science-fiction film as we saw city streets empty and gyms, restaurants, pubs, shops and cinemas close. Sports in every form came to a sudden halt. As people retreated behind closed doors to socially distance, poor mental health became an issue, even for many who hadn't experienced it before. I wanted to reach out and help people who might be suffering from depression. I also needed a routine to keep my own sanity in check. The daily live training sessions I did on Instagram with Paris and sometimes my five kids (if they were behaving!) ensured I started the day off on a positive note. I hope these workouts also helped others do the same. How many times I've banged my skull on that bloody chandelier in our front room while doing burpees doesn't bear thinking about, but the thought that we've been a catalyst for others getting fit and feeling mentally stronger for it gives me no end of pleasure. In fact, it got me to thinking about what else I could do. The road back to health was a tough and at times lonely one for me after my dark depression in 2015, but it was not without precious learning milestones along the way.

Sometimes, we get lost in the speed of life, and in the pursuit of our ambitions, and we lose sight of the really important things we should be thankful for, like friends, loved ones and our health. When you lose your happiness, your health declines, and when your health declines, it's game over. My road to redemption began with exercise and positive thinking. It's up to us whether we live our lives as glass-half-empty or glass-half-full people; whether we obsess over what's gone wrong in the past and what might go wrong again, or whether we look for a positive in every situation, however challenging. The quality of our thinking informs everything we do from the moment we get up in the morning to whether we get up at all. Being a fat, lazy bum with millions in the bank is no way to live, but being hungry, fit and really alive in the middle of life's journey, now that's a thing worth fighting for!

In years to come we might remember the Covid-19 lockdowns as a time the world stood still and gave us a chance to reflect on who we were, what we were grateful for and things we wanted to change. I believe you can take positives out of every negative, and the virtue of lockdown for me has been that I have been able to spend valuable time with my family. If we could remove the tragedy of the pandemic, perhaps we should have a few weeks' lockdown every year? Every morning as I look out from the balcony of our house at the nearby sea, I count my blessings. They say your life is a reflection of what you hold inside of you, and these days I'm glad to say it is light not darkness.

Before we begin, I want to give you four pieces of advice: short-term goals, positive thinking, healthy diet and exercise. Together, these are my magic formula. But 'magic formula' doesn't sound very boxing, does it? How about: this is my Furious Method. And you can follow it too. So today is your day – a day for change, a day to motivate yourself. You can do anything you put your mind to, remember that. Put the sacrifice and dedication in, and try to become a better person than you were yesterday. Be positive, spread good vibes and do great things. Now come on, you big dosser, let's get to it!

Tyson Fury

GETTING KNOCKED DOWN: HITTING ROCK BOTTOM

FURIOUS WORKOUT 1

Good morning, dosser. We're on it, let's go! This is a gentle workout to ease into things. Warning: they get harder.

1 Minute 30 Second Warm-up

(You can set timers on your phone or you could use an interval timer app)

- Jog on the spot doing straight punches with both arms for 20 sec
- Bounce on the spot for 20 sec
- Swivel hips clockwise for 10 sec, then the opposite way for 10 sec
- Slow squats for 20 sec
  (Stand with your feet hip-width apart, put your arms out in front of you and slowly lower yourself until your thighs are parallel with the ground – as if you are sitting on an invisible chair – putting weight on your heels. Then stand up straight. This is one rep)
- Kick legs out and shake for 10 sec

10 Minute Session

(Remember: hydrate and rest for 30 sec after each exercise)

- Walking lunges x 10
  (Lunge forward with your left leg and then your right. This is one rep)
- Jump squats x 10
  (Follow the same instructions for a slow squat, but faster, and jump up off the ground as you stand up)
- Press-ups/push-ups x 10
- Full sit-ups x 10
  (Lie on your back with knees raised and feet planted. Place hands behind head and use your abs to sit fully upright. This is one rep)
- Bicycle crunches x 10
  (Lie on your back, hands behind head. Lift left knee towards chest and bring right elbow towards left knee, while extending

right leg. You should feel a crunch across your stomach as you
partially sit up. Repeat for opposite leg/elbow. This is one rep)

- Star jumps x 10
- Half sit-ups/stomach crunches x 10
- (Like the full sit-up, but only lift yourself half as high off the
ground with your abs)
- Fast squats x 10
- Static leg lunges x 10
(Instead of walking forward with the lunge, plant left leg and
lunge backwards with right leg until left thigh is parallel with
the ground. Then alternate legs. This is one rep)
- Burpees x 10
(From standing, bend down and put hands on floor in front of
you, quickly kick both feet back behind you so you're in a press-
up position and then quickly jump feet back towards hands.
Stand up straight and then jump. That is one rep)

Warm-down

- Toe touches x 10 (standing – reach down as far as you can)
- Still standing, cross legs and slowly touch toes x 2, coming up
gently, vertebra by vertebra
- Roll hips x 5 each direction

If there was just one word I could give you to carry
forward and keep in your pocket for the rest of your
life, it wouldn't be 'diet', 'heart', 'courage', 'self-belief',
'commitment' or 'stamina' – though all are paramount.
It would be a ten-letter word that is the fuel for life's
greatest achievements: P-O-S-I-T-I-V-I-T-Y. Having a
positive mindset is essential in everything we do, and

the good news is that we have more control over our thoughts than we might realise. First thing in the morning, before my mind has a chance to come up with an excuse, I fly out of bed like a rocket and make sure I start with a positive act, which in my case is training. I go into it knowing that exercise will make me feel good straight afterwards, and that it is my daily medicine for life.

And, on that subject, let me just explain the exercises you'll find at the start of each chapter. I thought to myself, 'Wouldn't it be great if the reader could do a decent cardio workout and get fit by the close of the last page?' With that in mind, I invite you and your belly, and maybe even your family and your kids, to try these cardio sessions every morning. They'll start quite easy, but they'll gradually build to an almighty beasting! If you want to do the exercises every other day rather than daily, that's fine; try and build up at your own pace. It's not a race, my friend; exercise is a way of life. So, spend a few days getting used to Furious Workout 1 before moving on to number two.

If you've got your sweat on, now let's begin. Like any story worth its salt, mine begins with the main character getting knocked down. I believe we are exactly where we're meant to be at any one time, and that things happen to us for a reason. Boxing history is littered with tales of dark descents, of those who lost their way when the bright lights and the trappings of success disappeared, but few fighters have managed to come back from such a fall as me. I believe I was supposed to fall in such a spectacular fashion in order to make people sit up and listen to the pressing issue of mental health. I put this down to God's will; it was a battle I had to fight and continue to do so on a daily basis. Now, I don't want to dwell too much on the depths of despair I found myself in – this book centres on coming out of the dark and making the best of yourself. But those of you who haven't read my autobiography, *Behind the Mask*, need to know just how far I fell, if you want to appreciate the return of this Lancashire phoenix.

As 2015 drew to a close, I found myself in the hollowed-out, emotionally dead place Winston Churchill used to refer to as 'the black dog' of depression. And it wasn't just England's greatest Prime Minister who was periodically haunted by it; some of history's brightest comedians, actors, singers, writers and even astronauts have been carried off in its jaws.

I've known something was wrong with me my whole life. Growing up with my family, I'd often feel a loneliness even when I was with other people. I felt left behind. In 2016, I was diagnosed with bipolar disorder (previously known as manic depression) and obsessive compulsive disorder, and it was a massive relief to finally hear that there *was* something wrong with me, that it wasn't all just in my mind. Now I had a label I could apply to the way I felt; there were books about it, studies by famous neuroscientists. I wasn't mad, after all.

If you've seen that Jack Nicholson film *As Good as It Gets*, where the character he plays can't bear to stand on the cracks of the pavement (or sidewalk for our American friends), you'll have been introduced to the weird world of OCD (obsessive compulsive disorder). There are four types of OCD. In my case I have a thing about tidiness and wanting everything to be in order and in its right place. In fact, if something is amiss and non-symmetrical, be it a stranger's tie or a picture frame off-kilter, I have to politely intervene and straighten things up, otherwise it bothers me no end. The advantage of being almost seven feet tall is that no one has hit me for it . . . *yet*.

During my blackest days of depression, I would wake up first thing in the morning with tears in my eyes before I'd even sat up in bed. I felt as vulnerable as a child. Nothing seemed possible or worth doing; even boxing was about as appealing to me as yesterday's fish and chips leftovers. I had no energy for the three kids I had back then (now I've got five), no zeal for exercise, no vim . . . in fact, there was nothing left in my tank. We are only as bright as the fire that burns inside us and mine had almost gone out for good.

When I experienced my first ever panic attack, I went to A&E convinced I was dying from a cardiac arrest. It was the most terrifying experience I've ever had. I even told the nurse I thought I had been drugged with anthrax. My whole body was wracked with terror; I didn't know what was happening to me. As the saying goes, the greatest fear is fear itself. The unknown is more terrifying than the known and I was falling down a very frightening rabbit hole of madness. I hope to God I never have another of those mental assaults, but at least if I do I'll know what's happening. Knowledge really is power.

So, you might ask, what led to my full breakdown? Let me ask you a question in return. What do you do when you reach the top of the mountain you've always dreamed of ascending? There are dangers in getting what you've always wished for. Ever since my early teens I'd focused solely on becoming the world heavyweight champion; and not just a boxer, but the most skilful, light-footed craftsman among the giants since Muhammad Ali, then Cassius Clay, felled Sonny Liston. I danced and 'Ali shuffled' my way up the boxing ranks with one destination in mind: the summit. When I finally fulfilled my dream at the age of twenty-seven and took all of Wladimir Klitschko's belts, rather than being the moment I'd always waited for, it was a terrible anti-climax. Maybe you know what I'm talking about. Maybe you set yourself the goal of getting your dream job, or running your own company, or winning your local football or netball league. Then you put everything into that goal and after all your grit and hard work you succeeded in realising it. I wonder, did you give yourself a proper moment to soak it all in, to recognise the magnitude of your achievement? It's important to give yourself a pat on the back and give yourself credit when it's deserved. If not, you can feel hollow and directionless. Which is what I was like.

Were there any peaks left for me to climb after Klitschko? I'd achieved everything I set out to do and boxed everyone worth boxing. Instead of eyeing up my next challenge all I could see was a void, and without a fresh purpose to keep me going I came to a grinding halt. Depression can make life seem worse than it is, and in my mind I didn't feel I had anything to live for. There I was in the big empty. I was doubting everything and I prayed for death on a daily basis. Buying a Ferrari and having a few million quid in the bank should have been more fun than it was, but there was no substance to it. Nothing was of value. I wanted an appointment with the reaper, and feeling fed up with sitting in death's waiting room, I took matters into my own hands to speed up the process.

Within a month of being crowned world heavyweight champ I was an emotional wreck, on my way to a heart-attack thanks to a diet of Class A drugs, junk food and alcohol. As I had stopped training, my weight ballooned to 28 stone, and my mental health and marriage were both hanging by a thread. Everything I previously despised – including drugs – I now did; that's how much I had come to loathe myself. Until then I'd never taken my eyes off being a decent father to my kids, nor had I taken cocaine, and yet here I was keeping the cartels of Colombia afloat while also trying to drink myself to a very early grave. Drinking masks the pain while you're doing it but when you wake up in the morning you're even more depressed than when you started. Each day it was like having an angel on one shoulder and a devil on the other; one telling me I was good, the other that I was bad, worthless and that the world would be a better place without Tyson Fury. I didn't much believe in the angel. How quick we are to condemn ourselves and agree with the negative voices.

One day in June 2016, behind the wheel of my new red Ferrari, I thought I could switch off the pain and end it for good. As I sped towards the side of a bridge spanning the motorway, the Italian car doing 160mph, at the very last moment a voice inside my head said: 'Think about your kids, Tyson, your boys and girls growing up without a father.' And I thank God that I escaped the jaws of

27

despair. What stirred within me seconds before potential death was the very essence of life; I didn't want to give up. It was this small glimmer of light in the darkness that would start me on my comeback. If you have experienced suicidal thoughts I urge you to seek professional help immediately so that you can start your comeback too.

. . .

In one form or another, we will all get knocked down in life. Some of us will also know what it feels like to truly hit rock bottom. Repeatedly. But no matter how far you fall, and how awful it may feel, in my experience you have two lifelines available to you: one is hope and the other is gratitude.

You were born to enjoy your days; hope and joy at what is to come are hardwired into your system. Sadly, so too is fear, which can create anxiety and self-doubt, and can lead to despair. Every day of your life, hope and despair may be at each other's throats, and sometimes despair and the black dog of depression will win. My hope with this book is that I can show you how I've learnt to stop feeding my dog of fear and depression with juicy steaks, and instead to focus on hope getting a good run in the sunshine.

In my mind, focusing on happiness and positive things is the only way to achieve what you want out of life. It allows you to enjoy the journey, not just the destination. If you say to yourself, 'I'll be complete when I have a Porsche 911 in my drive', or 'When I become company director and smash the £100k salary then I can relax', I think you're kidding yourself. While goal-setting is central to making the most of yourself, don't betray today for tomorrow. If I told you we all had five minutes left to live before the planet turned to toast, what would your 'now' look like? Are you doing what you love at this moment? Are you with people you respect and that respect you? Do your loved ones know how much you adore them? You can improve the quality of your 'now' as soon as you choose to. This is where gratitude comes in. If you start living in the present, you will fully feel the force of gratitude for what you have.

Although we have fear in our DNA as a survival instinct, we weren't born to be scared and cowering versions of ourselves. People who manage their fear and are content in themselves don't let the negative talk in their heads dominate. They've learnt to be eagle-eyed and on the look-out for any destructive thoughts. I believe that when we control the flow of negativity we're letting into our minds, there is truly no limit to what we can achieve. The freedom of living in the moment is so powerful.

I also want to say that if you have depression, you are not alone. Depression has been documented as far back as the Babylonians and the ancient Egyptians – I'll bet you didn't realise I was a bit of a history buff! – and was seen as a kind of spiritual possession by demons. Gentle attempts to cure it included severe beating, drowning, locking in chains and starvation. The ancient Greeks and Romans were a bit more level-headed; they treated it with gymnastics, baths, specialised diets and calming music. Later still, in the ninth century, the Persians handled depression with water therapy and positive rewards for good behaviour. Throughout history other cures have included bloodletting and burning at the stake, and as recently as Victorian times, they'd throw you into an asylum and toss away the key for what in today's society are extremely common afflictions.

If you have mental health problems in the Travellers community you're not seen as a man, you have to hide it. My father suffered from depression. He told me: 'When I felt depressed I hid it from my family, so I'd not look weak. The pressure of being depressed as a young man with a family was almost too much. I was never in denial, I always accepted it. I used to take myself outside to a heavy bag in the shed, which I'd hammer for an hour. Then I'd go for a run, or walk the dog to try and straighten my mind out, get my ducks in a row . . . I'd tell myself I didn't want to feel like this and fix a smile to my face. Like you, Tyson, I used to ease my mind through exercise.'

Depression runs in the family. My dad told me that his dad was his mentor and used to suffer from depression too. My grandfather could read my dad like a book. He would say, 'Sit down and have a cup of tea, John.' Then they'd talk about old times and my dad would leave him ten minutes later with a genuine smile and feeling better.

Believe me, depression is more prevalent than you might think. According to the Mental Health Foundation, in any given week one in six of us in the UK is hit by depression or acute anxiety; one in five of us has considered suicide. It's important that we keep talking about it.

Speaking personally, I know that bipolar disorder's manic highs and deep slumps will never leave me of their own accord; I'm stuck with the shadow of depression for the rest of my life. For many people, bipolar can be tamed by taking regular medication. Check with your doctor as it may be the best thing for you. For me, one of the things that consistently keeps depression at bay is regular exercise, as well as a fixed routine and ensuring I have a sense of purpose to my days. When I say I use exercise as my medicine, I'm talking about knackering myself out a number of times per day, so that when my head hits the pillow in the evening I'm straight off to the land of nod. These days my depression is muzzled and walks beside me on a very short tether; I don't let it off the leash. Although over the years many people have told me that the most important thing we have in life is our health, I've only recently realised the full truth of this advice. Without your health, it's so much harder to enjoy the natural treasures of everyday living. With your mental and physical health, you're already wealthy. If you're reading this book and making the most of your days despite mental and physical impediments, you're one of life's warriors and I salute you.

Recently, I seem to have become an unofficial ambassador for mental health in sport, and it's an honour. I'm here to inspire and help others and I want to reassure everyone that there is light at the end of the tunnel. It takes a depressive to know one. I can often tell if someone is suffering depression right away, as their body language can tell a story: little eye contact and hunched shoulders, as if the person is trying to make themselves small and invisible so nobody will see them. That's how it feels on a dark day, even for a giant.

My friend Ricky Hatton bravely opened up to the media about his battle with depression, on World Mental Health Day last year. He said: 'It's very hard to describe it unless you've been there yourself. It's just totally depressed, no motivation, not the will to even get up in the morning. You know you need help, but you don't want to tell anyone. You're in bed crying every day.'

Sometimes I'll see a stranger who looks fed up and I

just wander over and give them a hug. It's my intention to smash the stigma of mental health; surely if the two-time heavyweight champ of the world can talk openly about battling depression, then others can too. I now use the stage I've been given to do good things and, where I can, try to make people happier. I fight to give the oppressed, the depressed, the alcoholics and drug addicts hope every day, so when they wake up in the morning, they know there's someone out there banging a drum for them. Being a depressive addict is like wilfully pulling the pin out of a grenade over a family lunch and letting it detonate everything that you love and value: your family, friendships, hard-earned security, your reputation and lust for life. Nobody is mentally ill for the fun of it.

I live on the edge and wear my heart on my sleeve. I've been straight down the barrel with people and told the truth about my mental-health struggles. For the first time, the British public have begun to get a sense of the real me and what I've been through. Before, I was a performing monkey for the promoters, and I was sick of it. The boxing community constantly expected an outlandish performance from me and it was exhausting, and becoming bad for my mental health. With the comeback I've had a chance to present the real Tyson. And I still have fun!

I hope that whatever fall and knockdown you've had in your own life, your comeback will present you with a fresh opportunity like I've had. You too can show the world the real you. You too can turn your worst negative into an enormous positive. After all, if I can do what I've done, and come back from where I've been, nothing is impossible. If you're at rock bottom, remember two lifelines: hope and gratitude. Use them so that you can start again, and become even better than you were before.

GETTING BACK UP: BUILDING RESILIENCE

FURIOUS WORKOUT II

Good morning, warrior. You're looking handsome and beautiful today!

1 Minute 30 Second Warm-up

- Jog on the spot doing punches with both arms for 20 sec
- Bounce on the spot for 20 sec
- Swivel hips clockwise for 10 sec, then the opposite way for 10 sec
- Star jumps for 20 sec
- Kick legs out and shake for 10 sec

15 Minute Session

(Remember: hydrate and rest for 30 sec after each exercise)

- Walking lunges x 15
- Jump squats x 15
- Press-ups x 12
- Sit-ups x 13
- Bicycle sit-ups x 13
- Half sit-ups/stomach crunches x 14
- Squats x 13
- Leg lunges x 13
- Burpees x 12
- Left jab, straight right, left uppercut (left foot forward, right foot back) x 15 (then swap: right jab, straight left, right uppercut, with right foot forward, left foot back)

Warm-down

- Sit on floor, legs straight out, touch toes
- On floor, one leg straight, one leg bent, touch toes for 10 sec then switch leg
- On floor, back straight, feet back and pressed together, push thighs down for 10 sec
- Standing up, pull one knee up holding foot with hand, feel burn in thigh, switch leg
- Rotate hips for 30 sec then switch in other direction

Rocky Balboa once said (yes, I know he's not real!): 'It ain't about how hard you hit, it's about how hard you can get hit and keep moving forward.' He's not just talking about boxing, either. He's talking resilience, defined as the ability to adapt in the face of change, trauma, adversity and stress; to bounce back and keep going; to never give up. Sly Stallone knew a thing or two himself about not giving up. In fact, the journey from writing the *Rocky* screenplay to the film making it to the big screen is in many ways an analogy for Rocky himself.

Long before the *Rocky* franchise earned more than $1 billion, Sly Stallone was a struggling actor with a slurred voice he'd had since birth and an acting career that couldn't even catch a cold, never mind a break. He'd had – legend has it – eighty-odd auditions and not scored one single job. Stallone was living semi-rough, his sometime house an oversized sheepskin coat he slept in. He'd sleep in bus stations and rent impoverished rooms where he said they had hot and cold cockroaches. He went from audition to audition and was getting nowhere. But he didn't give up on acting, even though it seemed to have given up on him. It got so bad financially that one night he had to make a choice: he could either feed his new wife and himself, or their dog, Butkus. Stallone was forced to sell his beloved bullmastiff for $40 to a short man with an attitude outside a 7-Eleven.

Soon after, Stallone had an audition with a couple of producers for a film. True to form, he wasn't right for the role, but as he was leaving, his hand on the door handle, he said: 'I write too.' He told them the outline of *Rocky* – they didn't know it wasn't actually written yet, but the idea had been in his mind ever since he saw a journeyman boxer called Chuck Wepner go fifteen rounds with Ali in 1975, even knocking Ali down in the ninth round before being knocked out himself – and the producers said they wanted a look at the script. Sly went away and wrote *Rocky* in just three days. The producers loved it and made an offer of $100,000 for the script. You might think that's the happy ending, now get on with the rest of the book, Tyson. But bear with me . . .

Given that Sly had barely $100 to his name, the $100k offer was a fortune, the first taste of sweet triumph in what had been a life of dejection and rejection. Stallone had worked every menial job possible (including one cleaning lions' cages) in order to survive. He agreed with the fee on the basis the producers allowed him to play the lead role. They had other ideas: Burt Reynolds was one, as was Ryan O'Neal, who'd done a little boxing as an amateur. Sly said no, it was him in the role or nobody, and the offers went up and up. Though they offered him over $200k, he held out for the lesser offer of $70k, but with him still in the lead role.

He hadn't forgotten about his four-legged friend. Sly found the man he'd sold Butkus to and asked to buy him back, to which the reply was, 'Sure you can have him . . . for three thousand bucks.' In the end the man agreed to a part in the film and is in the opening scene.

What should we take from this? When you work hard at something and invest yourself in it, no matter what the odds against you might be, never lose hope and belief in yourself. Who could have predicted that night outside the 7-Eleven when he watched his dog wander away with a stranger that Stallone's films would go on to make over $4 billion? He's a survivor who is pure resilience; he couldn't get an acting job so he wrote a role for himself. Never give up, there's a *Rocky* and a Sly inside all of us.

Being resilient is about having a sufficiently clear idea of what you want to achieve, so that whatever life throws at you, you will get back on course, however long it takes, however thick the fog, and reach your desired destination. A resilient person rolls with the punches and keeps moving forward because he or she has a purpose, a reason for doing it. If we don't have a strong sense of *why*, we let ourselves off the hook when the going gets tough and opt for an easy life. We remain in our comfort zone, a place where we're not stretching ourselves or evolving. You have to have a good reason to push yourself through hell – otherwise what is the point of getting burnt?

Resilience isn't just about being knocked down and getting back up, though. It's accepting that change is an unavoidable part of life and that the sooner we understand this the better. While we can't control the problems life unexpectedly presents us with, we *can* control how we choose to react to those problems: either with calm grace and quiet positivity, or throwing our toys out of the pram and sulking.

The person who has a strong enough *why* can tolerate almost any *what*. The first step towards developing resilience is focusing on your *why*. Why is it important to you and who will it help? Once I decided on my *why* – being a good husband and father again and winning back my title so I could help people with similar problems to myself – I had a sense of purpose that I believed in and suddenly, my life became infused with meaning. It was like a calling, a mission.

Throughout the course of the pandemic, with government restrictions designed to slow the spread of the virus proving difficult, the resilient businesses were those who were prepared to adapt to survive, whereas the companies sticking with the old models of doing things were shutting down every day. The *why* of the survivor is to keep going and weather the *whats*, be they the Covid-19 storm, or a short rude man outside 7-Eleven who walks off with your dog.

Deciding to carry on living and not hit that bridge at the last second was where I found my *why* again: it was my family. I realised how precious they were to me, what a gift life is and that it should never be squandered. Every day is a blessing and if we could only realise it, we have the freedom to achieve anything we want. The only thing standing in our way is ourselves.

My business is boxing, it's my job. I love it and I know nothing else. After my breakdown, I decided it was time to return to work. Only now I had a different engine powering me, a different *why*; it wasn't for the pomp and glory this time. From now on I wanted to use my celebrity to attract attention to the plight of those with mental health issues. If I was going to preach about mental health, then I needed to show the world I was a credible and active advocate, and that recovery was possible; it was time to walk the talk.

Having dragged myself out of the pit of despair, I agreed to the first fight with Wilder. I was still 27 stone. That might seem extraordinary to you, but I was so fixed on my goal and so sure that the Gypsy King could do it, that even the sight of a large pot-bellied man looking back at me in the mirror could not deter me. I could still dance lightly on my feet even at this heavy weight, and when I sparred my skills and boxing IQ were there, it was just my fitness and weight that were lacking.

When my first date with the Bronze Bomber arrived, 1 December 2018, I was far from ready both mentally and physically, but I knew I had the smarts to prevail. I believe in destiny and this gave me the courage after three years out of the ring to take on the biggest puncher in the history of the sport. When I was knocked down in the twelfth round, I lay there on the canvas and thought to myself, 'This isn't over. This is not how it ends.' So I got back up and took the fight to Wilder.

People all over the world have been intrigued by my comeback journey, particularly my refusal to give up after being pulverised by that right hand of Wilder's. It inspired people in a way I could never have predicted, and its message was simple: when life knocks you down you *can* pick yourself up again and come back. Only you can decide to do this, but in getting to that point you should welcome the support of others.

Part of what helped me build the resilience to get up again was the support of my loved ones and friends and the team around me. I truly believe that we have nothing to lose by being honest about our weaknesses in life with those closest to us. In fact, it makes us stronger, as we're no longer hiding something that's weighing us down. On the other hand, we have everything to lose by keeping our failings held in; we live in the shadows dragging our dirty secret around with us everywhere we go. That's no way to live. If you share your shortcomings with others, and their reaction is less than supportive, then you know you're spending time with the wrong people. I'm glad to say that most people around me have always been very encouraging when I have confided in them.

I keep a very small circle of family and friends around me in general. I admit that I'm not very good at making new friends. This is partly because in my position some people are interested in hanging on to my coat-tails. But my family and friends have been so key to my comeback, which is an important lesson. Remember, you don't have to do everything on your own. Find your own team; find who fans your flame, rather than dampens it. They're probably already there; sometimes it's about recognising the people who are already fighting in your corner (we'll come back to this subject a bit later in the book).

• • •

Hope, having a purpose and developing resilience to achieve my goals have been key ingredients to the success of my comeback. My wife, Paris, quickly noted the difference in my behaviour once I'd figured this out: 'Tyson was always depressed, either moping or partying, one extreme to the other. Then it finally clicked in his head; it was like a light bulb went on inside him, from darkness to light again. Everything went from "What's the point?" to him being happy, with a desire for life, all systems go; happy to live, to play with the kids or go for a walk. He got back into his exercise and he had a spark for his training.'

That's not to say I kept constantly on course during my comeback. There were hiccups along the way, relapses into negative moods. But I knew where I was headed and I held on to that co-ordinate and kept going, even when unforeseen things happened. In fact, I got comfortable with the fact that I had to be ready for the unexpected, personally and professionally. I had learned this lesson in boxing. A good fighter knows how to think on their feet and make changes to their style if a game plan isn't working, or something unexpected comes up like a sudden injury. When Joe Calzaghe defended his WBO super middleweight title against Evans Ashira in September 2005, he sustained a broken wrist and had to rely on only one hand for three-quarters of the fight to win the decision on points. Afterwards, Calzaghe said: 'I would have loved to have got a knockout, but a champion can adjust and that is what I did.' There's resilience for you. These days, thanks to being positive, having a goal (a *why*) and getting a lot of exercise, I no longer fear curveballs. I face them head on. I consider it as something to challenge me and make me grow. *What can I learn from this?* I ask myself.

Scar tissue is hard tissue that forms and hardens over a boxer's eyebrows when they get cut, and is much tougher than tender skin, making it more resilient to future blows. Maybe you lost someone you loved, you were made redundant, got divorced or became ill; sad as any such event is, you will have developed resilience as a result of surviving it. The way in which we respond to difficulties defines who we are. Resilient people accept that suffering is a part of life, and resist feeling sorry for themselves when bad things happen. Instead of asking, 'Why is this happening to me?' they recognise that everyone has tragedies and challenges thrown at them at some time or other.

There *are* ways to get through your darkest days. Battlers choose life, look for things to be grateful for and make a habit of being positive. It might be an old saying but there's plenty of truth in 'Count your blessings'. Humans are led by their thoughts and it's been scientifically proven that by practising gratitude and thinking of a couple of positive things every morning that you're grateful for, you can lower depression and increase happiness.

Part of my return to health involved learning to tune in to the good in and around me rather than punish myself for my weaknesses and shortcomings. My inner voice, instead of being destructive and counter-productive, had a bit more compassion for what I'd been through and I learnt to look at myself with more forgiveness, accepting that it would be a long road back to good health, and that I needed to take one day at a time, gradually edging towards my goal. Once I started to support, respect and like myself a bit more, positive things started happening and I began to attract good fortune. Positivity breeds positivity.

If we learn to look at adversity as an experience that we can learn and grow from, rather than a curse, difficult situations immediately feel different. They become challenges rather than brick walls. We're not born with in-built resilience; it's a mix of behaviours and actions that become habits to us when we change our way of looking at things. For example, I can look back at my mental breakdown and say, 'There goes three years of my life down the drain that I'll never get back,' or I can consider it as a period of darkness that led to the happier place I'm in now. Resilience starts with believing you can cope with any situation, no matter how challenging it is. What doesn't kill you might not make you physically stronger, but it will make you wiser, which in itself is a form of strength. The fighter who learns from his or her defeat and licks their wounds to return and fight another day has not lost everything.

Take Anthony Joshua, the poster boy of heavyweight

boxing. Contrary to all the rubbish written about what I supposedly think of him, I think he's done very well with his life and has come a long way from living in a council flat in Watford. He's a world-class athlete and a multimillionaire, who has made serious adjustments to himself since he had trouble with the law as a young man. The life he has created for his whole family is amazing. I respect that. I also respect that when he lost to Andy Ruiz, a small fat man with even bigger cheese pouches than me, in June 2019, AJ handled that defeat with the grace and humility of a champion. He had to ask himself some very serious questions. On the night he had produced a lacklustre performance. To his credit he made no excuses and went away and rebuilt himself. When he re-emerged for the sequel he was a different fighter and displayed better boxing IQ, and although he played things safe, using his jab and keeping Ruiz on the outside – just as Lennox Lewis did with Mike Tyson in 2002 – it was a good result.

The reason I mention this is that, at the worst time in his career, AJ showed resilience in how he chose to respond to the problem. Resilient people get to know themselves as a matter of necessity. They're more aware of their mindset than those people who blindly drift through life, and if they start experiencing negativity in themselves, they're good at spotting where it came from and weeding it out. They operate with a growth mindset; one that's not arrogant and presumes it knows everything, but one that is always looking to improve on itself. Resilient individuals are honest with themselves about their weaknesses and prepared to look at why they may be failing so they can address it and improve.

If we feel we're facing an insurmountable problem the best thing is not to let our emotions overwhelm us, but to stop and take a breath, coolly breaking the problem down into achievable chunks. You wouldn't rush into climbing Everest without listening to others' advice and experience, then carefully planning your route. You'd do your homework, make sure you had the necessary skills and equipment, and where there was a gap between your ability and what was required to succeed, you'd concentrate on those weak areas.

Winston Churchill once said: 'Success is the ability to go from one failure to another with no loss of enthusiasm.' Every storm, every failed attempt we survive and learn from makes us more resilient. Our true self is forged in the fire of adversity, that place where we get to know what we're really made of. Resilient people are also compassionate about the difficulties others are facing and at their best when they are helping people weaker than themselves. In doing so they take the focus away from themselves and place it on another. Ever since I've taken up the mantle for shining a light on mental-health problems, all that other glittery stuff – the Ferraris, Rolex watches – feels redundant, silly and a load of bollocks. That said, there's a lot to be said for owning a nineties Mini coupe . . . if only I could get in it. I should have gone to Specsavers.

THE COMEBACK KID: SETTING YOUR GOALS

FURIOUS WORKOUT III

How are you feeling today, ladies and gents? If you're feeling stiff, it's working!

2 Minute Warm-up
(You know the drill by now)

- Jog on the spot for 20 sec
- Toe touches x 10
- Cross legs, slowly touch toes (or reach as far as you can), 10 sec x 2
- Bounce on the spot for 20 sec
- Swivel hips for 20 sec, then opposite way for 20 sec
- Kick legs out and shake for 10 sec

15 Minute Session
(Remember, hydrate and rest for 30 seconds after each exercise)

- Walking lunges x 15
- Jump squats x 15
- Press-ups x 5
- Sit-ups x 15
- Bicycle sit-ups x 15
- Straight punches in front you (alternating arms), while running on the spot for 30 sec
- Half sit-ups/stomach crunches x 20
- Squats x 15
- Leg lunges x 15
- Burpees x 15

Warm-down
- Sit on the floor, legs straight out in front of you, touch your toes
- Still on floor, one leg straight, one leg bent back at the knee, touch toes for 10 sec then switch legs
- Plank position: lying down on your front on the floor, lift yourself up onto your forearms and elbows, keeping your tummy and legs off the ground with your toes touching the floor. Keeping your back flat, hold your abs in and stay off the ground for 20 sec
- Standing up, pull one knee up holding foot with hand, feel burn in thigh for 10 sec, then switch leg
- Rotate hips for 30 sec then switch in other direction

Keep Yourself Busy

In life, no matter where you start from, if you have a target then I believe that 99 per cent of the time you'll eventually hit that target. But if you don't have a target, then 100 per cent of the time you won't hit it – because there's nothing to hit! No matter how far away you are from your goal, you will get there if you persevere because you have a clear idea of your destination.

Someone once said, 'A goal without a plan is still a wish.' That's the difference between people who talk a good idea, and those who actually realise the idea. When there's a lack of planning or structure in your daily life, not only are you unlikely to achieve your goals, but you can allow negative thoughts into your mind. From there, it's easy for your mood to spiral downwards. We saw this during the Covid-19 lockdown, when some people who were used to having tasks at work were sent home and forced to go on furlough and await further instructions. Suddenly, millions of ordinarily industrious people in the UK no longer had their normal goals to define their day, and in some cases lost their sense of purpose. Some thrived on it, and took up new hobbies and set new goals. But others found it hard and panicked as if they'd been dropped in the middle of the sea with no sign of land to swim towards and nothing to hold on to. They started to experience anxiety, mental-health problems and in some cases even clinical depression.

This loss of purpose, and the problems associated with it, can happen to anyone, and it doesn't take a pandemic for the situation to arise. It's common when professional sportsmen and women retire, when soldiers finish a tour of duty, when office workers experience a redundancy, when the careers of teachers, doctors and nurses change suddenly. It can happen in fact to anyone whose days have previously been carved out with tasks. We can find ourselves lost and flailing for a sense of *self*. Speaking from my own experience, I tried retiring from boxing once, but I couldn't find anything that fulfilled me the way boxing did. I didn't know who I was.

The lesson I've learned is that whatever your potential, if you don't have a clear goal in life, a well-planned target to pursue, you'll sink. We all need goals to challenge ourselves and give us a sense of purpose; we are at our best when we're striving for something bigger than ourselves. That's why humans have evolved and thrived, otherwise we'd still be mucking about in trees flicking crap at each other. We're at our happiest when we are motivated, when we feel ourselves stretching and achieving rather than standing still. The word motivated originally meant 'moving cause'. Just like a rolling stone that doesn't gather moss because it's always moving, we should be the same. It's also a bit like boxing. If you keep moving, there's a better chance you won't get hit.

In this chapter I'm going to analyse some of the goals that I've set for myself in my career, so that these examples might help you create your own goals. But we're going to start with some strategies for goal-building, and how to see these goals through, as well as the pitfalls to avoid. So let's begin.

• • •

Clear Goals Make Better Lives

First things first, how do you create a goal and then break it down into achievable chunks? One top-line strategy to help you is based on an acronym called GROW, developed in the 1980s by business gurus Graham Alexander, Alan Fine and Sir John Whitmore. Maybe you've heard of it? It's used for coaching, and it's very straightforward.

G = Goal – your goal
R = Reality – current place in relation to your goal

O = Obstacles/options – possible approaches you might consider

W = Way forward – which/when

How it works in a nutshell: think of what your **goal** is. **Realistically** speaking, next ask yourself how far you are from achieving it. For example, if you have a marathon to train for, how many miles can you run at the moment? You then need to identify what are the potential **obstacles** to achieving your goal, and your **options** for resolving them. If you're training for the marathon, do you have a historic injury that will likely flare up, and what can be done to treat it? And finally, you need to figure out the **way forward** – *which* option are you going to use first and *when* will you do this?

When you think about what your goal is, my first piece of advice is to have a *very* clear goal: be as specific as possible. You *must* be able to measure success, otherwise it's harder to judge if you actually achieve your goal, and you'll be wasting precious energy in areas you don't need to. In Hollywood they say a good film idea is one that has a great 'elevator pitch': a film you can pitch in a single sentence, during a short ride in a lift for example. In the same way, your goal should be a simple sentence of intent and personalised so it belongs only to you: 'I, Tyson Fury, will be an ambassador for mental health.' That's a start, but it's still a bit vague, and vagueness is for dossers. It's more powerful if you can make your goal time-specific, because you'll not be able to wriggle out of it. For example, 'By the end of 2020 I, Tyson Fury, will be an ambassador for mental health and will have set up my own foundation for the Morecambe community.'

A helpful way of remembering this thought is a quote from Greg S. Reid, a motivational speaker, entrepreneur and author of the book *Wealth Made Easy*:

'A **DREAM** written down with a date becomes a **GOAL**.'

It's equally important that it's your goal, and not someone else's. If the goal originates with someone else, the goal's potency is diluted, and there's less chance of you digging your heels in and being resilient when obstacles occur. Ultimately, you're more likely to lose interest and fail when you're following someone else's goal or dream. But when the goal comes from you, there is a sense of ownership, and the ups and downs you suffer en route to achieving it are bearable because you know it will be worth it.

Be sure to make your goal a hard one too – dare to dream big. My mindset is always, *I'm going to be the best or nothing else*. I refuse to be second, third or fourth. I became heavyweight champion of the world because I refused to even consider settling for anything less. There is no 'can't' in my vocabulary.

The Importance of Visualisation

My next piece of advice is to make your goal one that you have to really think hard about how you are going to achieve, so that you can then start getting excited about the process. Ask yourself, what positive impact will it have on your life and those around you? It's about making your dream into a goal and talking to yourself and maybe others regularly about it so that it becomes *real* to you. At some point, somewhere in your subconscious, a handshake takes place between your body and mind as they agree to work together towards achieving it. If I had a pound for every time I've told people I was going to be the future champ of the world, I would have undoubtedly earned far more than I already have.

I recommend giving your imagination a bit of exercise and picture the feeling of succeeding in your goal. I'm not a massive visualiser, in so far as I don't – unlike some people – imagine every little detail about where I want to get to. With me, it's a broad co-ordinate; I fix the destination of my goal in my mind and then give 200 per cent in getting there.

There's a lovely little story about Jim Carrey practising visualisation at the start of his career back in 1987, when he was broke and only had a few dollars to his name.

Every evening he'd go up to Mulholland Drive, in the Hollywood Hills, and sit in his car staring down at the lights of Tinseltown. He'd imagine directors telling him they liked his work and he would visualise good movies coming his way. He believed he had these jobs and contacts already but they just hadn't found their way to him yet. He took his visualisation to the next level when he wrote a cheque to himself for $10 million for 'Acting Services Rendered' and carried it around wherever he went. He gave himself five years to achieve this payday in real life. Just as the cheque – by now moth-eared – was about to disintegrate, Carrey was paid $10 million for appearing in *Dumb and Dumber*. As it happened he was only a year out: it took six years to achieve not five.

Muhammad Ali, who you'll realise by now is one of my favourite boxers, also believed in visualisation. He said: 'It's the repetition of affirmations that leads to belief. And once that belief becomes a deep conviction, things begin to happen.' He also said: 'I am the greatest, I said this even before I knew I was . . . I figured if I said it enough, that I would convince the world that I really was the greatest.' If your mind can see it and believe it, it's a lot easier to achieve it. We write our own stories with belief, sweat, blood and dreams.

I'm a great believer in destiny, but I think it is helped on its way by the strong intentions of an individual. Some say 'what's for you won't pass you', but if you think fortune will come and knock on your door while you happily do nothing, then you're going to be disappointed. You still need to strive to make your dream happen. If I believe in something 100 per cent I can will it to happen. I think about the dream until it becomes reality. I think it through again and again, constantly imagining it happening. I can convince myself that the most impossible things are possible. I remember that after just one phone call to Paris – and I wasn't even going out with her at the time – I told her that she was going to fall in love with me and that we would get married and have lots of children. I knew what I wanted from a young age and I willed it all to happen. I knew I wanted to be heavyweight champion of the world and I knew how to go about it, as if it was all laid out clearly before me. It wasn't easy but I thought about it every day and my goal became a reality. As a boxer coming up through the ranks I used to tell myself: 'This is you. This is your time, your era. These men are no good to you.' More recently, I wanted to go and crack America like all the greats in music and sports do. Sure enough, I got the Top Rank deal and I went on to conquer America. I was convinced it was all down to destiny and pure will on my part. And it was. It all became true.

Once upon a time there was an undefeated three-headed monster in the heavyweight division – AJ, Wilder and the Gypsy King. Nowadays, at the time of writing, things have changed. I'm the only unbeaten champ left of the original three, and Oleksandr Usyk has arrived on the heavyweight scene with his victory over AJ. I always said I was a standalone fighter. Even when I was fighting Klitschko I knew it was written down by destiny that this was my time. The Chisoras, Joshuas, Wilders or Hayes are just names in my era. They will tell their grandkids one day how they lived during the reign of the Gypsy King; that they boxed Tyson Fury. Just like in the ancient world, when the Greeks spoke of how they fought in the era of Achilles.

Remember: **SEE** your **GOAL,** shape it, order it and **WILL** it to happen.

Focus on Your Immediate Challenge, Not Ones in the Distant Future

Although it's good to have lifelong dreams, you also need to think about the present. I focus on one day at a time as a building block to getting me nearer to my goal.

An example of this 'one day at a time' thinking is how I approach my fights. The British boxing press are always wetting their lips over the prospect of future fight(s) such as the Gypsy King versus Anthony Joshua for example, which has been talked about for years. Personally, I never visualise fighting someone far in the future as there is every chance it will never happen. And that applies to life in general. You have to take every opponent and situation very seriously, focus on what your next challenge is, not others further down the line.

· · ·

Once you have chosen your main goal, it's important to break it down into achievable, measurable mini-goals, which act as check points of progress as you gradually work towards your ultimate destination. Make sure these mini-goals are attainable, as with each one tackled you'll gather momentum and they will pump up your confidence. By all means push yourself, but know the difference between this and flogging yourself silly. If you punish your mind or body with too much too quickly it can cause long-term damage. So pace yourself, take baby steps and congratulate yourself on each step you've succeeded climbing up the staircase of your challenge.

Here's a method called the 'Goal Ring', which might

help you identify your main goal and all the smaller goals that will need to be ticked off if you're going to nail it.

The Goal Ring

Draw a square boxing ring, with four points for the four corners. In the middle of the ring write your ultimate goal, then in the top left corner write the first mini-goal on your journey. Working clockwise around the ring, in the second corner write your second mini-goal, and so on. By the time you get back to the top left corner, you should hopefully have broken your goal down into four manageable portions, in order of importance. Once you are happy with the ring, you can add the dates by which you want to have achieved each of the mini-goals.

○	○
1st Mini Goal	2nd Mini Goal
ULTIMATE GOAL	
4th Mini Goal	3rd Mini Goal
○	○

The Goal Scorecard

Another way of thinking about this is to draw a twelve-round scorecard, like in boxing. For each round, write a goal, and leave three columns: one to write a completion date, another to tick off whether you have achieved that goal, and a third to give yourself a mark out of ten, just as a judge would score a boxer. In this way, you form a record for your goals in life, similar to how a boxer has a record from a fight that they can reflect on and learn from.

GOAL	DEADLINE	COMPLETED	SCORE

My plan for getting back to mental wellbeing was partly achieved by giving myself short- and long-term goals related to my physical health, the first of which was to lose 180 pounds. I then broke this big goal down into smaller chunks, so that every ten pounds I reached I would give myself a reward – a nice day out with my family, a meal, some new clothes; it could have been anything really. These goals gave me a crucial thing to focus on and brought meaning to my days, which had become loose and endless. I started training twice a day, cardio work and boxing, and I took it gradually. When I signed up for the Wilder fight, I knew I had six months to get back into shape, and that timeline was motivating. I was taking a risk but by setting goals and working hard I lifted myself out of depression and learnt to appreciate life again.

Another goal that I broke down into smaller, more manageable portions occurred during my second fight with Wilder. Because our first match was a draw, I knew that if I wanted to guarantee becoming heavyweight champion of the world in our rematch, I would have to change my approach, because it's hard to get a boxing decision by points in America. So my fresh goal for the second Wilder fight was to win via knockout. I wanted to go for broke and overcome him with more aggressive tactics. I had my goal, now I needed to break it down into a series of steps, the first of which was to find the right coach to bring that aggression out of me. Historically, I'm a slick boxer, not a mauler or a streetfighter, but to win via knockout against a warrior like Wilder, I'd need to really step up my brutality.

Steve 'Daddy' Bunce is probably the most respected boxing journalist working in the UK today. Like myself, he identified that I needed to be more assertive with Wilder if I was going to beat him second time around, but cautioned I shouldn't be *too* aggressive. I needed to get three or four inches closer to Wilder, then detonate my own right fist but it would put me right into the danger zone of Wilder's fearsome punches. Bunce said I needed to respect my opponent the same way I had in our last encounter and remember how dangerous he still was. As Wilder himself likes to say, 'My opponents have to be alert and on top of it for thirty-six minutes, while I just need to be lucky for two seconds to land [a punch].'

While I fully respected the danger his fists presented and worked towards defusing it at my training camp, come the night I didn't want to respect him at all in the ring. I wanted to intimidate and bully him with his own style.

I decided to hire Javan 'SugarHill' Steward, nephew of the late, great Manny Steward, who started the famous Kronk dynasty in 1970s Detroit. I'd met SugarHill ten years before when I turned up at the gym unannounced and got on so well with his uncle Manny that he let me live at his house for a month while I trained with him. SugarHill is very gifted in his own right. The next mini-goal was getting ready with some tune-up fights to get me comfortable in the ring again, followed by training camp and the fight itself; all of them separate endeavours leading to one destination.

Every boxer, and indeed every person in life, you meet has different strengths and weaknesses. For the second Wilder fight my team and I focused on creating a new habit of hitting a 250kg heavy bag with concussive punches. Rather than tapping and moving around it, I was smacking it so brutally that it was regularly knocked off its hook. I've never focused on landing these kinds of shots before as that style of fighting is not my cup of tea, but with practice they became second nature.

When fight night came around, all of the plans and mini-goals in my quest to knock out Wilder came together with spectacular results. With the focus on the power shot plus my decision to cramp him with my extra weight (we'll come on to that later in the book) I was able to bully Wilder in a way he had never been experienced before, constantly putting him on the back foot, so he was going backwards much of the time, a direction he isn't used to going in. Forget the boxing result or the tactics for a moment, the lesson here is this: if I'd skipped any of my crucial preparatory stages on the way to my goal, and gone in without a plan, it would have been a very different story.

Remember this little equation:

STRATEGY + EXECUTION = REALITY

. . .

Overcoming Naysayers to Reach Your Goals

There's a pretty good chance your successful goals will be matched by a few failures, and there will certainly be obstacles to realising every goal you set yourself. But don't let these setbacks or hurdles limit your dreams. Humankind can do anything it puts its mind to: it has created fire, the telescope, split the atom, built supersonic jets, transplanted faces, and even put a man on the moon. You need to remember that you are part of this incredible species, and have your own gifts that you can bring to it. Don't let anybody tell you that you can't achieve your goals or dreams. You can. It's my dream to go to space as one of the first space tourists and I'm already focusing on this and making it happen.

I see myself unstrapping myself from a comfy chair and floating through the cabin of a spaceship to stare through a large window in awe of the beautiful blue place we call home.

Muhammad Ali once said: 'Impossible is just a big word thrown around by small men who find it easier to live in the world they've been given than to explore the power they have to change it. Impossible is not a fact. It's an opinion. Impossible is not a declaration. It's a dare. Impossible is potential. Impossible is temporary. Impossible is nothing.'

What a man Ali was, and what a thought that is. People are achieving their true goals all the time, every day. Who is to say that you can't be one of them? Often it can be those close to us who make us doubt ourselves because they want to guide us to take the safe route, the well-travelled path through life. But for some of us that's not what we're after. I wanted to become the undisputed world heavyweight champion and, with 7.4 billion people on the planet, realising that dream was never going to be child's play. So I say, don't think about the odds, they mean nothing. Wilder was odds-on favourite to knock me out the first time we met and look what happened. The dosser had written me off when he saw a photo of me looking like a middle-aged cream puff with a hangover, and I came back and schooled him.

My dad, once a very good boxer himself, didn't really encourage me to box as a lad as he knew the risks and didn't want me getting hurt. People said: 'You want to become heavyweight champ, Tyson? You'll have to fight huge men.' My response was: 'Well, I'll just have to be huge as well.' Whatever it took, I was determined to get there. I was inspired by the words of another fighter too. Bruce Lee once said, when talking about obstacles that can get in the way of achieving our goals: 'Be water my friend.' In other words, be fluid so you can flow around or through the obstacle and thereby beat it.

Remember: *anything* is possible. I saw an inspiring video on YouTube of a teenager skateboarding, doing some amazing tricks. But this particular kid is blind and uses a stick to feel the way in front of him. Instead of obsessing about how difficult this approach would be to master, he focused on how much he wanted to achieve his tricks. You see, your mind can conquer extraordinary things if you focus on the end product, rather than let the challenges overwhelm you.

Elon Musk, the maverick genius behind PayPal and Tesla cars, was laughed at when he announced that his new company, SpaceX, has its sights set on Mars. He even gave a date of 2030. People said: 'Impossible. Too expensive. There's no rocket that can land on the red planet and then take off again and return to Earth.' So what did Musk do?

He designed one. And who knows, he might just do it. The sky isn't the limit for this fella, nor is space.

Life is too short for regrets. What we did yesterday is not important, neither is tomorrow. Live for today and be thankful for what you have. We need to unleash our potential to achieve our dreams if we're to live a fulfilled life, so if you feel like you haven't got a challenge, sit yourself down and crack on with the Goal Clock. Remember, happy people are goal-oriented people and unhappy people are stay-in-bed dossers!

• • •

Seeing Goals Through

Once you possess a clear goal, you'll feel a sense of purpose which you can channel your energy and effort towards. A person with a plan is dangerous. In the pursuit and execution of your goal you'll know you are on track to somewhere meaningful, not wandering blindly through life without a compass. Keep asking yourself, what is important to you and where do you want to go?

It won't be easy. But no CEO, Oscar winner, Formula One star, artist, boxer, Olympic and Paralympic gold medallist ever achieved their goals overnight. Instead, they took a series of steps over a period of time to get to the next level. And it involved resilience, patience and blood, sweat and tears (quite literally in my case). Nobody starts at the top; you start at the bottom, you do your time, you learn your craft or business through your mistakes and you work your way up. Like we said in the last chapter, you learn through adversity; anything worth doing is hard to achieve and requires grit, otherwise everyone would be doing it. You have to give everything your best shot and sweat the small stuff, which means focusing on doing things thoroughly. You can never be satisfied that you know everything; there is always more to discover. And you must never settle for average; always strive to be the best at what you want to do. If you're doing what you love, often it won't feel like work.

When I began my comeback, most of the British public and the sporting world had written me off as a casualty, which was fine. I've always drawn power from others' doubts in me. I looked beyond the bloated thing in the mirror and focused on stepping back into the skin of the Gypsy King, persevering every day against the doubts bouncing around in my skull: could I do this again and was boxing was still for me? Did I have the dedication to lose the weight? My whole life has been a struggle with mental health and weight gain. I'd lost seven stone before, but losing ten stone was an altogether different matter.

Could I muster the right mindset? It was a hell of a demand to make on myself in such a short space of time. But I never lost sight of my goals during my comeback.

Aside from focus, grit and determination, another crucial quality to possess in seeing your goals through is being willing and flexible enough to change your goals when you have to. When the UK went into the first lockdown in March 2020, I, like many, had to rethink my goals and create some new ones. I knew that I wanted to keep my family safe away from the virus, to keep myself sane, and to carry on training and maintaining my fitness. At the same time I wanted to help others who were mentally struggling with self-isolating and social distancing. How could I reconcile all of this? The answer was to make daily videos of myself and Paris working out with cardio sessions and post them on Instagram. It was like my digital journal every day, checking in with people who follow me on that platform and bringing some sunshine to their mornings while taking them through their paces.

I never expected it to catch on to such a degree as it did. I started getting messages from people all over the world saying how much they looked forward to the morning sessions, how it was helping them maintain mental resilience and how much they appreciated me being honest about my struggles with depression. It felt like a big family we were all a part of and I realised there are so many people in the world like me who are suffering with mental health and that these people need a gee-up every day.

It's vital to make new goals all the time to keep you engaged and present. Look what happened to me when I finally achieved my dream of beating Wladimir Klitschko and taking his crown. I was lost because I hadn't planned *beyond* that moment. After the two Wilder fights it was different. Mentally, I knew myself so much better after what I'd been through, and now I was aware how vital a part exercise played in keeping the black dog at bay. So make sure you plan for the moment beyond your goal; get ready to find a new goal for when the time comes.

YOUR FURIOUS GOAL

To finish this round, I want you to think of a major goal you would like to achieve in your life but that you haven't allowed yourself the opportunity to tackle yet. The more challenging and life-changing the goal the better. Let your imagination stretch its wings and give yourself the freedom to think big.

Write it down here (remember: it should be a single sentence).

GOAL:

_____

_____

When do you want to achieve it by?

_____

_____

What resources do you need to help you achieve it? (These resources can be personal and practical)

_____

_____

_____

What if any obstacles might stand in your way?

_____

_____

_____

What resources/capability do you have to respond to these obstacles?

_____

_____

_____

Life Values and Priorities

Specific, measurable goals are important. Equally important are fundamental lifetime values and priorities that are not as easy to track the progress of, but are vital as codes to live by, and which help you aspire to be better. These are what we are going to briefly explore now at the end of this round. I understand we live in a world where we have to work to pay our mortgage or rent, settle the bills and put food on the table, but nobody said you have to be miserable while doing it. If you're in a dead-end job that you don't care for, you're never going to be happy and you're not going to achieve your potential. Also, you're better than that. Who is to say you can't do something else you really love and get paid for it? Nobody. Nobody worth listening to anyway.

Make your own mistakes – then no one is to blame but you. If you're following your dream and it doesn't work out, at least you've tried. What's that saying, 'Better to have loved and lost than to never have loved at all'? Well, better to have tried and given your dream goal your best shot then never to have tried at all. So many people at the end of their lives confess on their deathbeds that they wished they had taken more risks in their life. You've got to follow your heart, your gut feeling. Change your job if you're not happy; only you can make it happen. If you've got a goal and you're passionate about achieving it, then one day you will reach it, but only if you start to turn the dream into a goal and map it out, otherwise it will remain just that: a dream. And if you have no dreams then you're going to be in that dead-end job until the day you die and you're going to be very unhappy. Do what makes you smile; life is too short to be miserable.

At some stage in your life you have to come clean and stop kidding yourself, accepting who and what you are, because you can soul-search all of your life and time waits for no one. These days, through the lie of social media and reality TV, people get sucked into the sparkly dream of celebrity: jewels, mansions and champagne, turquoise swimming pools and snow-white sandy beaches . . . with worshipping fans at every corner. I say: don't think about being famous for the sake of being famous. Follow your passion and consider who will benefit from it. I've never put material things in front of what really matters to me: my craft of boxing and my family. I could live in a twenty-five-room castle if I wanted to but I don't need the space. I live in a five-bedroom house in Morecambe, Lancashire with my wife and our five kids and we have what we need.

The Three Most Important Things in Life

These will vary for everyone. But I believe we should all hold important values, and try to live by them. For me, I'd say the three most important things you can have in life are good health, a loving family and being happy in your own skin.

1. Health

As I've said before, your health (both physical and mental) *is* your wealth and is foremost. If you do have health problems, hard as they are, try to consider that things could be a lot worse, and to remember that people who look like they have everything going for them on the outside most likely have their own problems and crosses to bear; we just can't see these issues as obviously. Poor health limits us but with resilience we can cherish the remaining health we have and our attitude towards our illness.

One of my most inspiring pals is a guy named Shaun Gash, who I met in 2017 on the long road of my comeback. A car crash twenty years ago left him with a broken back, punctured lungs and cracked ribs. He woke up paralysed from the waist down and wheelchair-bound at the age of nineteen. Shaun's take on life is that things happen, obstacles come your way and it's how you deal with them that counts. He also believes that every cloud has a silver lining, and he's living proof; at the spinal rehab unit where he was recovering, he met his future wife Dawn, who worked there as a nurse. We all have different things to overcome, and these challenges are what make us who we are. Shaun's mindset is: *Do I let them make or break me?* The accident hasn't weakened him, if anything it's made him stronger. He's been in a chair for twenty-nine years now and he says: 'I wouldn't change anything. I've scuba-dived, climbed Ben Nevis, Snowdon and Kilimanjaro. I don't think I would have done half the things I've done without the accident happening.'

He fully accepts his paralysis but instead of feeling sorry for himself, his affirmation is: *The chair is me and I am the chair.* His kids call him Poppa Wheels. Others around town in Morecambe call him the Wheelchair Adventurer, or the Daredevil in the Wheelchair. And just as I have tried to break down social barriers around mental-health issues, Shaun takes delight in rebooting people's perceptions of the disabled so they say to themselves: 'He's in a wheelchair but it hasn't stopped him from doing anything.'

Recently, he was scaling Ben Nevis when his leg was crushed and he had to have it amputated. I saw him on the Thursday and he told me he was off to hospital to have his leg chopped off. I then bumped into him back in the gym on Saturday. I couldn't believe it; he'd discharged himself on the Friday! Did he moan and feel sorry for himself? Despite having been in a wheelchair half his life, he is as positive as a man who has won ten gold medals. We cheer each other up when one of us is flat and push each other on. At the start of every week we send each other a 'Monday Motivator', something by text which is positive and starts us off in the right frame of mind. We also send a 'Midweek Kick' and a 'Friday Feeling'.

With all that Shaun has going on he is still an incredibly positive person. And he makes me think: 'If he can have such a positive effect on me, why can't I do the same for others?' Shaun believes that if you can make a difference to even one person, that's a great thing. He's an amazing character and one of the nicest people you could meet; always organising stuff for charity and helping others out. Things happen, obstacles come your way and it's how you deal with them that counts. We all have different crosses to bear, and it's these that make us who we are. Shaun has also taught me to only worry about things that you can control and to put the rest out of your mind.

2. Family

My family are the driving force behind everything I do. I'll come back to my family and my friends later in the book to do them justice, because having a loving family is the most important life goal anyone can aim for. Why did I make my comeback from depression? My family. Why did I get back up from the dead when I was out cold in the twelfth round against Wilder? My family. Why do WWE wrestling? OK, I confess I've enjoyed watching it since I was a child. But it was the joy my children get from it that ultimately made me do it. For them to see their dad taking on Braun Strowman made me feel so proud.

3. Happy In Your Skin

Being happy and comfortable with who you are is my third most important big goal in life. If you work in McDonald's and are content then you're already a spiritual millionaire. If you're at peace with yourself and enjoy what you're doing, you are *so* much more successful and wealthy than billionaires who spend empty money chasing material pleasures but still find themselves wanting and lost. Believe me, I've met these spiritually bankrupt wallies and they're ten-a-penny. It's a fool's game they play: they can never enjoy what they've achieved because they're too busy worrying what the next person is worth. Me, I'd rather be on the dole living in a council flat and happy with my mental health, than living in a mega mansion and getting down all the time. When you've tasted the dirt at the bottom of the pit, you realise that nothing is more important than knowing and valuing yourself and those closest to you.

If you're not happy with yourself, put in the work needed to become who you want to be. The writer Ernest Hemingway, a keen boxer himself, once said: 'There is nothing noble about being superior to your fellow men. True nobility lies in being superior to your former self.' We can always improve who we are. I'm not suggesting you pretend to be someone else, but if there's an aspect of yourself you want to change in the long term, like becoming more disciplined with exercise, or standing up and speaking out at work or in your personal life, only you can make it happen.

BACK YOURSELF (EVEN WHEN OTHERS DON'T)

FURIOUS WORKOUT IV

Good morning! Right, let's crack on.

1 Minute 30 Second Warm-up

- Jog on the spot for 20 sec
- Bounce on the spot for 20 sec
- Swivel hips for 10 sec, then the opposite way for 10 sec
- Kick legs out and shake for 10 sec
- Punches on the spot for 10 sec
- Star jumps for 10 sec

Leg & Tummy Workout

(After each set, rest for 30 sec, hydrate and then do a second set. Take your time. It's not about the speed, but about the quality of your form in each exercise during this workout)

- With a dumbbell in each hand (choose a weight you can comfortably hold) perform 10 squats, 2 sets
- Walking lunges x 20, 2 sets, pushing back off your front leg
- Jump squats x 10, 2 sets
- Press-ups x 10, 2 sets
- Sit-ups x 20, 2 sets
- Burpees x 20, 2 sets

Warm-down

- Toe touches x 10
- Cross legs, slowly touch toes x 2, coming up vertebra by vertebra
- Roll hips x 5 in each direction

The Louisville Lip

Fear and self-doubt are the nervous lapdogs of failure. Self-confidence is about trusting in your ability to achieve your goals and desires and knowing your worth. When you watch early footage of Muhammad Ali (then Cassius Clay), one of the first things that strikes you about him is the force of conviction he has in himself. That and his extraordinary talent and charisma. He barely pauses for breath during his pre-fight interviews about how he's going to beat his opponents, firing out the same sentences repetitively until they become mantras. No wonder the press dubbed him the 'Louisville Lip'! But just as Ali knew that pre-fight trash talk was part of the psychological warfare of professional boxing, he also knew a thing or two about self-realisation; namely that if you say something enough times, to enough people – including your opponent! – they start to be hypnotised or spooked and begin to believe it, and before you know it, your beliefs become true.

In 1964 Ali had his first shot at the world heavyweight title, against Sonny Liston, and the odds had him a 7/1 underdog. Leading up to the fight, Ali's constant flow of self-promotion and rhyming soundbites mystified Liston, an ex-thug enforcer with ties to the mob, who had been in prison and liked to let his fists do the talking in the ring. He was scared of no one but had no idea how to deal with such an outspoken personality as Ali. For all Ali's confident jibes, most sportswriters thought Liston was going to kill him. Meanwhile, the leggy young kid from Kentucky predicted he would take Liston in the eighth round. 'Sonny might be great, but he will leave in eight,' Ali said. 'I'm young, I'm handsome, I'm fast, I'm pretty and I can't possibly be beat. If you like to lose your money, you bet on Sonny.' This continual verbal assault went so far as Ali gate-crashing Liston's training exhibition in front of the press and public.

Eventually the moment arrived when the bell rang and the world got to see if Ali could walk his talk and bring down the unshakeable Liston. He most definitely could. Dancing artfully around that canvas as gracefully as a matador, Ali peppered the bull-like Liston with rapier double jabs and won in the seventh round when the beaten champ refused to leave his corner. Throughout a professional career spanning sixty-one fights, Ali used a mixture of sorcery, personality, impossible natural skill and ring savvy to overpower, confound, confuse and wear down his opponents. But it was his tireless self-belief that was the most important part of his winning formula. Even towards the end of his career, it was a beautiful thing to watch him come to life as he summoned the confidence in himself and radiated it charismatically to others so they reflected it back to him. I'm not often lost for words myself and have been known to talk the hind legs off a donkey. I learnt this from watching the Louisville Lip. Maybe I should be called the Morecambe Mouth!

Never Question a Fortune Teller

When Joe Rogan interviewed Wilder on his podcast after our first fight, Wilder said he thought I'd put some kind of gypsy spell on him. As far as I know I don't possess much in the way of spells (though my Irish grandmother was a fortune teller). What's clear is that I got into his head and shook his self-confidence by repeatedly telling him I was going to drop him in the second round. I planted that seed in his mind and uttered it so frequently in the run-up to the fight that he got spooked and started believing it himself. All it takes is a seed. When my dad was just twelve years old my grandmother predicted that one of her grandsons would become world famous, and one would drown. Given that half of her prediction has come true, neither me nor my brothers are keen swimmers and will never go out of our depth if we can help it!

I believe some people have the ability to read the future. It's a gift that my people are open to and have practised for thousands of years, but if I was a scientific type I would say it just goes to show the seeds we plant in our head can work both ways, negatively or positively. Whether we believe in clairvoyance or not, we need to be constantly mindful of the seeds we plant for ourselves and ask ourselves whether they are beneficial and serving us or not.

We can create new self-beliefs in the same way we create positive habits. If you tell your brain enough times that you're good at something, it will become seeded in your subconscious and your unconscious actions will try to make it a reality. By our own design we can become *anything* we want to.

The Hardest Fight is Against Yourself

I remember the look on Ali's face after his first round against George Foreman in their famous 1974 meeting in Zaire, known as the 'Rumble in the Jungle'. As Ali returns to his corner after three minutes of toe-to-toe slugging with big George, he is clearly shocked by the brutality of Foreman's punches and knows the other man is too strong, too young for him to fight on the inside for fifteen rounds. Ali's face for a very brief

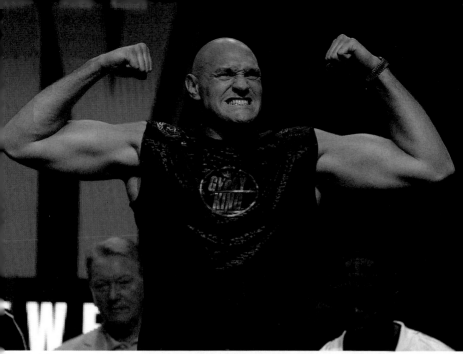

The night before Fury vs Wilder II, I weigh in at 19 stone 7 pounds (273 pounds), Wilder clocks in at 16 stone 7 pounds (231 pounds). Both of us are heavier than we were last time, but there's more to this game than weight. I'm in the shape of my life and I'm the master of mind games. I've already burrowed deep into Wilder's head. (Credits: *Al Bello / Getty*)

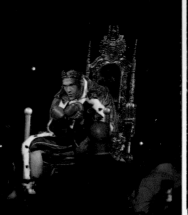

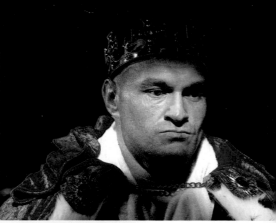

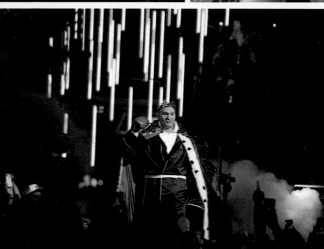

The Gypsy King has arrived! I always enjoy coming up with ideas for my ring walks; they're like my miniature productions. I pick songs and outfits that mean something to me and that people can relate to. For tonight's battle I'm dressed as a king in a crown and cape, sat on a golden throne and carried into the arena. I'm accompanied by the syrupy voice of Patsy Cline singing 'Crazy' – an ironic nod to my mental health battles! I'm ready for a twelve-round war or a one-round knock-out. It's my time to shine. (Credits *Al Bello / Getty;* top left and middle, *John W. McDonough / Getty*)

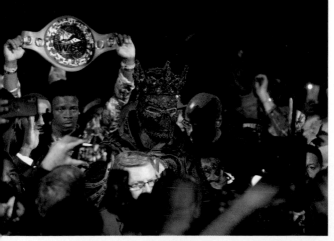

From a cloud of dry ice and beams of purple light emerges Wilder, also wearing a crown, and decked out in glittering black armour. True to form he's hiding behind another mask as he does for all his entrances, this one with glowing red eyes. He looks extraordinarily . . . daft. It has been fourteen months since me and the Bronze Bomber last 'danced' back in December 2018. Let's see if the dosser still calls me 'pillow fists' at the end of this fight!

(John W. McDonough / Getty)

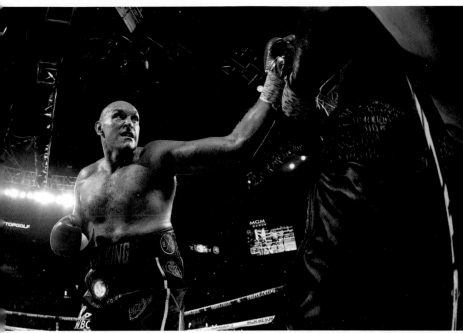

As the bell for Round One rings, I sprint out to the middle of the ring to control the action, working the feint and hitting the Bronze Bomber with solid spearing jabs. Towards the end of the third round, I hit Wilder with a quicksilver left-right hook combo, and literally whip him on to the canvas. (Credits: *Al Bello/Getty*)

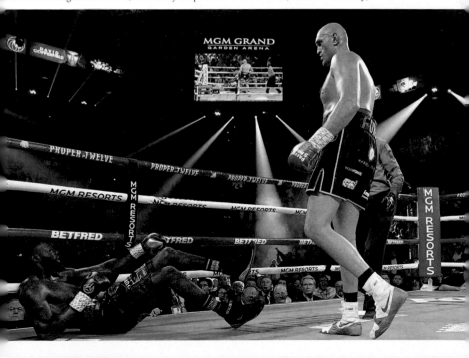

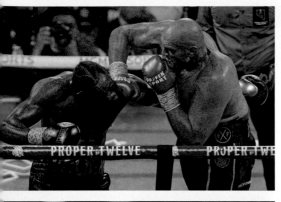

Top: I've been telling Wilder throughout the build-up to the fight that I'm going to be dropping my own bombs. Maybe he didn't believe me, but now that it's happening, Wilder seems surprised by the weight and power of my shots. (*John Gurzinski / Getty*)

Middle: Round Five and straight away I pepper Wilder with yet more jabs and some big overhead right hands, all of which connect. Wilder stumbles in the corner and clinches for want of something to lean on – and soon regrets it. Bad move, dosser. With the extra weight I'm carrying I'm able to wheel him around to wherever I want him.

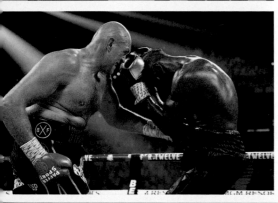

Below: Wilder is floppy as a ragdoll. The fire ha been gone from his belly ever since the end of the first round, but now he's markedly groggy, in the throes of defeat, his lip split, his ear a rose o blood. (Credits: *Al Bello / Getty,* middle & bottom)

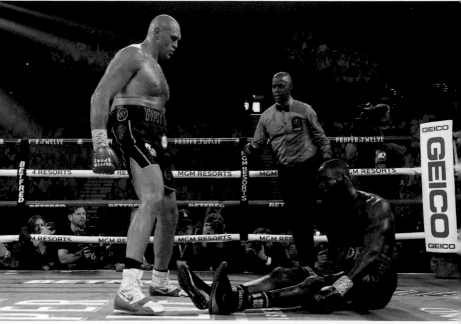

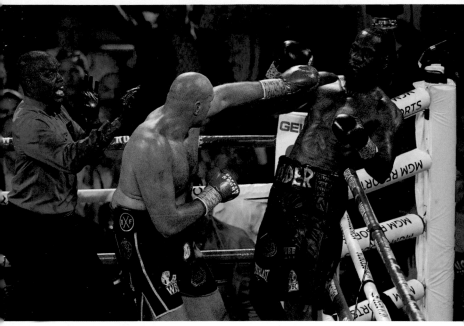

und Seven. I have Wilder pinned in the corner and am firing direct jabs like a nail gun; one after the other, they
erce his guard and find their target on his face. Another one-two combination, a body shot and then the crowd
pts as something white flies through the air. In his peripheral vision Kenny Bayless sees the towel land and wades
to stop the barrage of my punches. I don't remember a great deal else about the fight after this. So much adrenaline
s popping through my veins like champagne bubbles, it's hard to describe the euphoria.

edits: top, *Mark Ralston / Getty*; bottom left, *MB Media / Getty*; bottom right, *Al Bello / Getty*)

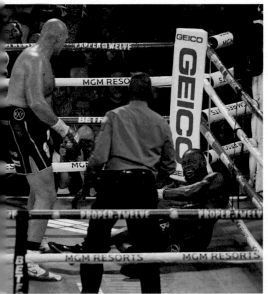

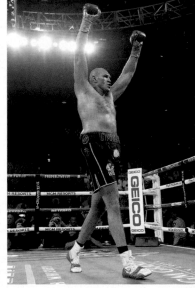

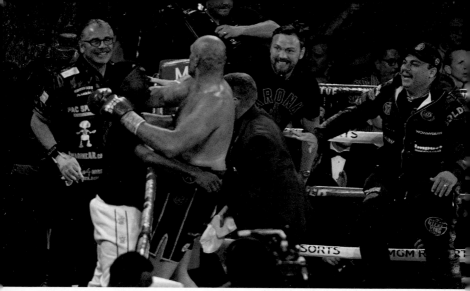

Celebrating with my team. I've just been declared the winner and here I am hugging my trainer SugarHill Steward. To nail this fight I channelled my aggression – and nobody does controlled aggression like SugarHill and the legendary Kronk Gym in Detroit. The battered heavy bags I destroyed and knocked off their hooks in training were evidence of the explosive style I'd been developing just for Wilder. The game plan went perfectly. (*MB Media / Getty*)

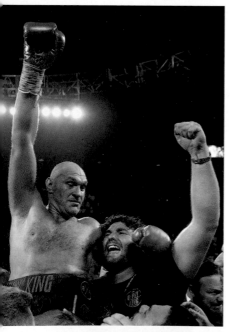

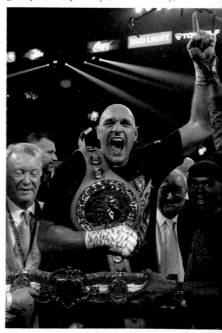

The crowd was mostly a blur as I was lifted up on my brother Shane's shoulders. Grateful to have him in my corner. (Credits: bottom left and right, *Al Bello / Getty*)

Me and my belts, alongside my UK promoter, Frank Warren (left), my US promoter, Bob Arum (right), and SugarHill Steward (far right).

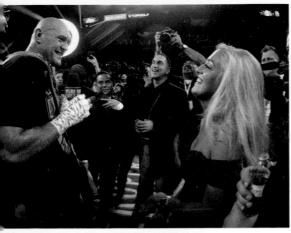

The morning after Halloween 2017, at my lowest point, I said to my wife, Paris: 'I'm on a mission to become the heavyweight champ again.' Three years later and Paris was ringside at the fight, dazzling in a ruby dress. Although she doesn't like watching my fights, she watched me definitively beat Wilder and take the WBC heavyweight title. Mission accomplished. I hugged Paris and my brothers and team. Together, we had done it. (Credits: top and middle, *Al Bello/Getty*)

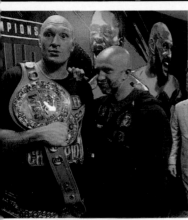

Middle: 'Old Baldy Head'. The nickname me and my strength and conditioning coach, Kristian Blacklock, have for each other. I met Kristian at the start of a training camp for my Klitschko fight back in 2015. I've kept with him ever since.

Below: With Team Fury, celebrating in Vegas after the win.

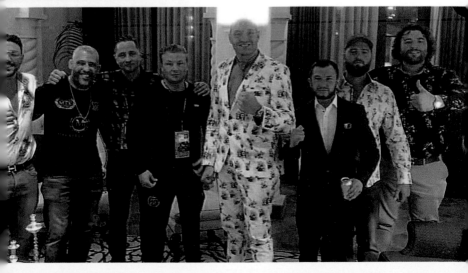

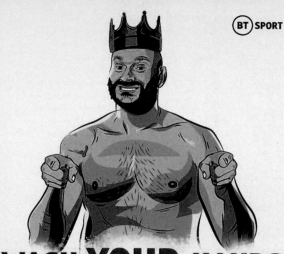

BT SPORT

WASH YOUR HANDS YOU DOSSERS

Top: What made me sit down and write this book? In March 2020, a global pandemic turned our lives into a science fiction film. Sports in every form came to a sudden halt, and I wanted to reach out and help people who might be suffering from depression. I also needed a routine to keep my own sanity in check.

Below left and right: The daily live training sessions I did on Instagram with Paris and sometimes my five kids (if they were behaving!) ensured I started the day off on a positive note. I hope the workouts also helped others do the same. I never expected them to catch on as much as they did! The thought that we've been a catalyst for others getting fit, and feeling mentally stronger as a result of it, gives me no end of pleasure.

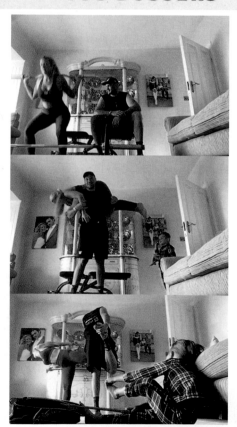

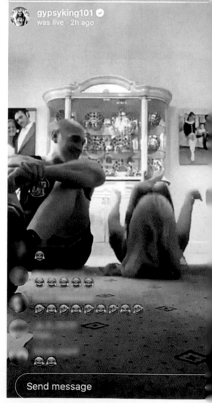

gypsyking101
was live · 2h ago

Send message

moment shifts like an emotional kaleidoscope through a moment of fear and desolation and then changes to self-mastery. It's as if he is reminding himself of that mantra he'd been teaching the crowd leading up to the bout: 'Ali bomaye.' *Ali kill him.*

Ali had been banned from boxing for three years after being convicted for draft evasion and was coming back from defeats at the hands of Joe Frazier and Ken Norton, not forgetting he was seven years older than Foreman. A little like Wilder when I faced him, Foreman had no losses and had won thirty-seven of his forty fights by knockout. Nobody believed Ali had a chance as it had taken him the full twelve rounds to beat Ken Norton in their rematch, while Foreman had turned off Norton's lights in two rounds. Similarly, Smokin' Joe Frazier had lasted only two rounds before Foreman ate him for breakfast. In short, the current heavyweight champ was a human wrecking machine.

Ali didn't flinch from the harsh reality that the younger man was stronger than him. All through his training camp at Deer Lake he had prepared using the rope-a-dope technique, which involved covering up against a boxer and leaning back on the ropes to absorb the power of the other's shots. Before their gloves touched for the start of the first round, Ali looked at Foreman and said: 'You've heard of me since you were young. You've been following me since you were a little boy. Now you must meet me, your master.' Ali supercharged his self-belief by drawing from the belief of the local Kinshasa crowd as well as drawing on his previous triumphs spanning decades of boxing.

You probably know the rest of the story – Ali used the rope-a-dope technique brilliantly and Foreman punched himself out. All the while Ali kept whispering in Foreman's ear, diminishing his resolve and self-belief, then took him apart in the eighth round. Ring savvy versus brute strength.

In my career I've certainly learnt from Ali. Admittedly, Ali didn't call his opponents dossers. But I definitely like to talk to my opponents in the ring, and do anything I can to play mind games with them. In the second Wilder fight, I wouldn't shut up talking to Wilder in each round. There had been so much talk in the build-up that he was going to draw blood from me and open up the cut above my eye that had been stitched up after my previous fight against Otto Wallin. It was a bit of fun that now I was drawing blood from him. But I think my running commentary was the nail in the coffin and the final insult for Wilder as by that point I was completely bossing the fight.

The Enemy Between Your Ears

A large part of achieving your goal is about breaking it down, preparing properly and following a strategy, but without self-belief to execute that strategy we soon come unstuck. Laird Hamilton is a veteran American surfer who has surfed more big waves than anyone alive. He was one of the first to tackle the quickest, strongest and largest wave in the Pacific, known as 'Jaws'. He has looked down an eighty-foot vertical wall of water and rode the wave to tell the tale. The following quote by Hamilton sums up for me how we must have faith in ourselves, for if we are going to face what seems impossible, then we'd better believe we can do it, even if no one else does: 'Make sure your enemy doesn't live between your own two ears.'

Self-belief is vital if you want to achieve anything. We're all too quick to doubt ourselves and forget past achievements which prove our capability. But by recalling them we can strengthen our self-belief. Think back through your life, starting from your early years up to the present – what big waves have you ridden? I want you to remember any really positive events where you surpassed your expectations of yourself. See if you can pick at least six examples and then make a note of them. That's important, as by writing them down you are directly sending a positive message to yourself, giving your mind a very clear idea of what excellence looks like and alerting your mind to the standard you expect it to aim for.

Get so familiar with these big waves that if I was to call you up and ask you to name the six you could easily rattle them off. Ask yourself why you were successful, what your attitude was like, and what you did to help yourself achieve these trophy moments. The more you can get to know how you best work as a person, the easier it is to avoid what doesn't work for you. And in moments of self-doubt, or when others put you down, all you have to do is remember some of these key successes in your life to prop you up and keep you positive. Every time you think negatively about what you can and can't do, doubting your ability, remind yourself of one of these triumphs, how it felt in that moment. Just the feeling of that earlier success will make you feel empowered and ready for your challenge.

Remember the movie *Men In Black*? And that scene where a human turns out to have a little alien in his head, operating the body from the cockpit of his brain? Imagine a mini you in the cockpit of your head, steering your thoughts towards things you want to achieve and having a level of self-mastery over your actions. Each time you slide back into automatic unconscious behaviour, that's because the mini you at the controls has fallen asleep.

Every time you exercise and get your heart going this sends the mini you what it needs to direct you. You also feed the mini you when you say something positive to yourself, when you sit down and plan your goals, when you practise gratitude morning and night, and when you eat, hydrate and sleep well; all these things make your mind feel good. The icing on the cake is helping other people as this fills your heart, and is a better feeling than all of the others put together, but we'll talk about that in the last round of the book. In order to be able to help others, you need first to help yourself by making sure you're as vital as you can possibly be.

Banishing Negative Naysayers

The negative opinions of others can often hold sway over us, even if they are outdated or perhaps were never true in the first place. All it takes is a couple of nasty comments delivered thoughtlessly in a matter of seconds, and it can, if you're not careful, affect you for years to come. If a teacher once said to you 'You'll never go far in life', every time something hasn't gone well for you there's a very good chance that comment will come back to haunt you via a little voice in your head that says: 'It's true after all. You've never gone far and you never will.' We then often look for evidence to add to the barbed comments, as if we're building a case against ourselves. The problem is that humans are very good at knocking themselves down and underestimating their worth. We find it much easier to believe an insult than take a compliment. Just as we're more likely to remember our failures than our moments of success. And when asked about our strengths, we find it harder to celebrate them than to describe our flaws, which we do all too readily.

Some of our greatest leaders in history doubted themselves before they achieved amazing things: Julius Caesar before he marched triumphantly through Rome; John F. Kennedy after the failure of the Bay of Pigs invasion. It's not self-doubt that defines us in life, as we all suffer it at times, it's whether we can convince ourselves to go beyond the doubt and the choke point and get on with the challenge – just like Ali did between the first and second round against not so gentle George.

Have You Got the Stones?

When somebody has faith in you and makes an encouraging remark, it can carry you a long way. The sentence 'I believe in you' can have an enormously positive impact. My dad often told me that I was going to be the world heavyweight champion one day and because he's a man of his word and principles, I believed everything he said. Manny Steward, trainer of countless world champions, from my cousin Andy Lee to Tommy Hearns and Lennox Lewis, once pointed to me and told Wladimir Klitschko (whose training camp we were present at): 'Tyson is the natural heir to the heavyweight throne.' That was ten years ago to this very year, and although Manny is no longer with us, his belief in me has never left me. These people we meet along the way, who recognise our potential and spur us on, are like stone markers in the fog, and we should maintain their memory so that we can draw on their words of encouragement when moments of self-doubt start to niggle away at us. On the subject of stones, Ali painted the names of his greatest opponents on boulders and placed them on the mountain road he used to run up at his training camp, just to remind him of his victories and strengthen his self-belief.

Boxing is a hard sport and though I've been in the 'Fancy' (the fight game) so long that climbing into the ring no longer scares me, at this level of concussive punching I could be leaving my wife a widow every time I step through the ropes, under the lights and onto that gladiatorial square of canvas. I say a prayer to God before every fight asking him to protect both fighters and send them home safe to their families at the end of the night. It requires 'minerals' to climb into thirty-six minutes of uncertainty, and though it's the most exciting time of my life and I feel more alive than at any other time, I'm under no illusions. Each time may be my last and battling that takes self-belief.

The Importance of Positive Self-talk

If you feel like you have a long way to travel to reach your ultimate goal, the first thing you have to do is start believing in yourself and observing the way your internal voice talks to you.

First up, stop being a critic and start being like a coach to yourself. If something goes wrong, always bring the coach out. Don't ever call yourself a 'loser' or a 'failure'; encourage yourself instead. Take care and be kind to yourself; charity starts at home, as they say, and you have to build yourself up before you can be of help to others. Treat yourself with integrity, the way you would have others treat you. Instead of looking for faults, try and find things you've done well alongside areas for development.

If you lack confidence, it's possible to replace limiting views of yourself and plant new ones which give you conviction in your capabilities and help you rise beyond the glass ceiling of what you thought you could achieve. What we think of ourselves is directly translated into the life we currently live. Think about it. Then feel it.

If I say to myself 'You're a disappointment to everybody', and just dwell on that sentence, I start to feel a heaviness come over me, as if it were true. Thoughts directly affect feelings. We really are only as good as the thoughts we put into ourselves. What negative messages are you allowing into your mind on a daily basis? Each time one arrives, forcibly replace it with a positive thought about yourself. Try this: get an elastic band and put it on your wrist. Each time you experience a negative thought that diminishes your self-belief, pull it so it snaps back and stings you. To start with, your wrist will be sore, but gradually you'll input less of the unhealthy stuff into your mind.

In life, we unconsciously repeat patterns of behaviour and the only way to change these patterns is by altering our beliefs of ourselves. Neurologists reckon 95 per cent of our everyday actions are automatic, that's to say they are driven entirely by our subconscious mind and we do them without thinking. Most beliefs are embedded in us between the ages of one and six when, like sponges, we soak up our parents' beliefs, which were handed down to them by their own parents. Without this stored data of our experiences, beliefs and second-hand opinions we wouldn't have frames of reference to refer to when we make important decisions throughout the day. Our subconscious mind makes decisions on our behalf based on the info it can dredge up from previous experiences. It will look into the past to find the nearest approximation to what we're confronted by now. Even if the historic example is not relevant it will still use it rather than come back with nothing. The problem is that many of the beliefs the mind drags up are obsolete and no longer belong in the present; they're like old skin that we need to shed.

We Are What We Believe

What we believe is what we end up with. Albert Einstein once said: 'If you always do what you've always done, you'll always get what you've always got.' It's time to spring clean your head and bring in fresh, positive thoughts that challenge the thinking which holds you back. Have you ever noticed how quickly a negative thought can sprout at the back of your mind and then spiral you into a negative mood? Sometimes it's like our mind is against us, especially when we're tired or have had something go wrong. When this happens we need to step out of ourselves and ask, 'Is that thinking true?' or, 'Is this train of thought helping me or holding me back?'

When I was 28 stone, given the state I was in and my severe lack of self-esteem, it was hard to imagine my return to form as a world champion. I had to dig deep, reminding myself that I'd boxed since I was in my early teens, had never been beaten as a pro fighter and was still the lineal heavyweight champion of the world. And even despite this overwhelming evidence in my corner, removing the negative self-beliefs I had developed was difficult. To transform myself to the Tyson I wanted to be I had to see myself in the change and believe it; I had to keep reminding myself that the Gypsy King had never been affected by any of Tyson Fury's personal problems. For while Tyson Fury is a husband, father, son, brother, cousin, an everyday person who can be brought down by anything, the Gypsy King has never faltered, never lacked confidence in his ability and is untouchable. But I still wouldn't let him in my house. Would you!?

USE YOUR CORNER: ASKING FOR HELP & BUILDING A SUPPORT NETWORK

FURIOUS WORKOUT V

Good morning, gorgeous. Let's get sweaty!

1 Minute 30 Second Warm-up

- Jog on the spot for 20 sec
- Bounce on the spot for 20 sec
- Swivel hips for 10 sec, then the opposite way for 10 sec
- Kick legs out and shake for 10 sec
- Punches on the spot for 10 sec
- Star jumps for 10 sec

15 Minute Session

(Remember: hydrate and rest for 30 sec after each exercise. If you need longer to get your breath, take your time)

- Walking lunges x 25
- Jump squats x 25
- Press-ups x 15
- Sit-ups x 25
- Bicycle sit-ups x 25
- Half sit-ups/stomach crunches x 25
- Squats x 25
- Leg lunges x 25
- Burpees x 25
- Jogging on the spot: left straight punch, right straight punch x 30

Warm-down

- Sit on floor with legs straight out, touch toes
- On floor, one leg straight, one leg in, touch toes for 10 sec then switch leg
- On floor, back straight, feet back and pressed together, push thighs down for 10 sec
- Standing up, pull one knee up holding foot with hand for 10 sec, feel burn in thigh, then switch leg
- Rotate hips for 30 sec then switch in other direction

Society needs to reframe the way it views depression and recognise that it is a strong person, not a weak one, who reaches out for the help of others. That person has decided that they want to fight ill mental health and take care of themselves and their loved ones, but they can't do it alone. If this is you, I want you to be very clear with yourself – you're not pathetic, nor are you a failure; you're a life warrior, a torchbearer and a survivor. In this round, you'll learn the steps I used to get myself better and the order in which I used them.

Step One: Accepting You Need Help and Reaching Out For It

If you had a car with a leaking oil tank that was making the pistons seize up, would you carry on driving it till the big end ripped through the engine, or would you get it seen to? You don't need to wait until you're a casualty on life's hard shoulder. There are mental mechanics who, if you're willing to allow them, will assist you to get back up and running smoothly and happily again. Anyone suffering with mental-health issues, I appeal to you to reach out immediately and get professional medical advice. The sooner you do that, the sooner you can return to a normal life. I am not an expert and there is help out there, you just have to ask for it (at the back of this book I have listed a few organisations who may be useful too, once you have spoken to your doctor or GP).

To use a different analogy, the mind needs a good shepherd to guide it through difficult times; without one it lays itself open to attack from negativity. We have no idea just how powerful our mind can be, nor do we really appreciate its ability to direct the body to heal itself. For example, take the placebo effect. A patient is given a pill or treatment and told that it will make them better, when unbeknown to them there's nothing in the pill at all. Often patients record positive results despite the pill being a placebo, and these successful effects are entirely down to their minds and bodies. This illustrates the brilliance of our design by our maker. Every second we're alive our body is working hard for us, renewing dead cells and repairing itself as we sleep.

When you make the decision that things not only need to change but *have* to change, that is a key milestone in a return to your better self. It doesn't solve everything there and then, but it allows you to start thinking of what *good* might look like beyond the edge of your dark cloud. After I decided my next big fight was against depression, I still felt weak and vulnerable but now I was willing to be led by others until I was strong enough to be my own shepherd again. I went and got help from a leading psychiatrist.

During my recovery I also put my trust in my faith. I had my epiphany in a pub on Halloween night in 2017, hopelessly overweight and humiliated, wearing a badly fitting skeleton outfit that was skin-tight and emphasised my full 28 stone. I wrote about some of this in my autobiography. Although I had started training again, I was still drinking and going on benders and making life a misery for my wife, my children and those who were closest to me. Looking around the pub at people half my age I felt like a disgrace, and I knew things had to change. I left the pub early for a change and later that night I stood in my bedroom in my underpants, fell on my knees and cried out to God to help me. Tears were running down my face. When I got back up, I knew the comeback was on because I was finally asking for God's help and being honest that I had a serious problem.

If you don't believe in a faith that's fine, but just admitting you have a problem is a key building block to getting you on the road to your recovery. An acceptance of your addiction and an acknowledgement that you need help to deal with it is actually the first step of Alcoholics Anonymous' 'Twelve Steps' recovery programme. My addictive behaviours went beyond just booze: I was also addicted to coke, and self-loathing. But when that moment finally comes and you tell yourself, *This time I want to change, and I'll accept the help of others*, that is the real start; when you are ready to open up. After the night of the skeleton, I went to see a therapist.

On the pastel walls of the psychiatrist's office were photos of his family. I sat in a comfy chair and just talked. After our first exchange the therapist was sufficiently concerned about me that he told my father I was an imminent suicide risk, and my faith alone wouldn't hold me back from killing myself. My dad's response was to keep such a close eye on me that I never had an opportunity to act on it; he slept in my house over the coming weeks and watched me like a hawk.

I kept going to see the therapist once a week. Even by my standards, I did a lot of talking on those Fridays! I was initially sceptical about going, but it was a really positive experience. I've never opened up like that to a stranger; it was like letting poison out of a wound and also refreshing to be listened to and understood by someone who knew exactly what I was going through. Just by sharing my weaknesses I loosened the hold that this horrible demon of depression had had on me all my life.

The sooner you get professional help, the sooner you can go back to normal and reclaim your life. To keep you in check and get you back on track when you slip, you also need your cornermen and women; a team of trusted friends or family members who will keep you balanced. I had Paris, Dad and my friend Dave Reay in particular, but there were many others too, including my former trainer Ben Davison. I will always be grateful for their help and support – and we'll come on to how to create that sort of network in more detail later in this round. It's also massively helpful to share your worries, relapses and triumphs with others who are also suffering mental-health issues but are trying to get better too. My dad and Ben could both share their own struggles with mental health, which made me feel like I wasn't alone.

One of depression's worst aspects is its slyness; it waits in the shadows until you're on your own then sets to work on you, isolating you from others, colouring your thoughts black with hopelessness and anxiety. Every time I ran or tried to go to the gym in the early dark days of my recovery I was full of fear; my body felt milky, sapped and unwilling, so I stopped doing the one thing that would have come to my rescue – EXERCISE! This sabotaging voice in my head said: 'This life is not for you any more. You don't need to exercise. What's the point?' I felt zapped, and despite my good intentions I didn't want to live. By late 2016 and early '17, I *really* hated boxing. If you'd offered me a room full of diamonds for a round in the ring, I wouldn't have accepted.

A support network of people who understand you

and have your back can spot when you're slipping into certain behaviours and help you do things that are good for you. Before you know it the sly bully starts to shrink before your eyes. Also, it's a huge relief to get your depression out in the open with people you can trust. These days I have a few friends in the public eye with mental-health problems and we talk openly about our depression. It's important to have people in your life that you can disclose things to rather than bottling it all up. When you try and keep a lid on mental illness, the pressure will grow stronger and stronger until eventually the lid bursts open and you find yourself deep into a mental breakdown. It doesn't need to come to that bursting point if you spot the depression first, acknowledge it and then find help. If reading this you're thinking, 'I'm OK, my black moods aren't that bad . . . I'll get over it,' ask yourself a couple of questions:

- Do I get little pleasure in doing little things?
- Do I feel down every day?
- Do I struggle to get to sleep and wake up refreshed?
- Do I feel constantly tired?
- Do I feel alive or as if I'm sleepwalking?
- When did I last really laugh?
- Do I have little appetite or eat excessively?

- Do I feel like a failure?
- Do I find it hard to concentrate reading a paper or watching TV?
- Do I think I'd be better off dead?

If the answer is predominantly *yes*, you're most likely depressed, my friend. Don't fight the truth, don't fight yourself, don't be a dosser, get it seen to. It may be something that can be solved with talking, or it may be deeper, with a root system that stretches all the way back to your childhood. If your answers were generally *no* to the questions above, then consider yourself very lucky to have that mental health.

So, the first step of my recovery began with the admission I had a problem, and as I've said, I then sought help and kept up that help as a routine. My next step after diagnosis was to change my environment.

Step Two: Environment – Find a Positive Place With Positive People

Your environment isn't just the place you live in, it's also about who you have around you and whether they contribute to your ill mental health, or impact on you in a positive way. When I was at my lowest point after my suicide attempt, I took myself and my family away from my beloved Morecambe; in my present state of mind it was like some haunted theme park where my addiction had rooted itself with booze, cocaine and shenanigans in the not-so-fun Funhouse. So, in December '16, we left and moved my caravan onto Dad's land in Styal, Cheshire, the place I had grown up. I started to rebuild the pieces by creating a no-negative environment.

Paris, me and the kids lived there with my dad for the next six months, and even my brothers came to stay. We focused on living every day as normally as possible. It was a great environment to rediscover the simple things that make life special: nature, trusted company, good food, laughter, sleep and even singing! Another environmental thorn I removed from my side was the media, and the same went for social media (see more on how to block out the negative effects of social media in Round Ten). Media and social media can be a toxic environment, and during this time in my recovery I stopped watching as much TV, ignored Twitter and didn't so much as look at a news stand. Immediately I felt a release. Again, it was about creating a perimeter fence that would keep out any bears bringing negativity with them.

I was also glad to get shot of the false sympathisers, the people who rubbed their hands with glee at my downfall but pretended concern. Them and the gawpers who just liked to stare at my life as if it was a car crash. It's funny but it sometimes seems there are more people who like to see a successful person fall rather than root for them, probably because it reminds them of their own lack of achievement and ambition.

If you are blessed with a close family as I've been, nothing can beat the security you feel with those who have always loved you unconditionally and always will. I had a great corner of trusted family members and they dropped everything to be with me. They didn't care how much money I had or whether I was still the Gypsy King or not – I could just be Tyson in their company; brother, son, father, and sometimes wounded child. Being left alone to be a normal person meant everything to me, though being left alone completely was out of the question. I needed and still need people. Some of us are loners by nature, but not me. I love the chatter, the company, the stories, the jokes, the songs, the music . . . I draw my strength from my family. They're not all brilliant at understanding mental health, or talking openly about emotions, but I wouldn't swap them for all the rock on Blackpool's North Pier.

Step Three: Building a Support Network

Limit your support network to your family or best friends; you don't need an army, just a few people who you trust 100 per cent. You know a best friend because they are always there for you and would do anything for you in times of trouble, and you'd do the same for them. I could call my best pal Dave at any time, for anything.

The secret is to keep your team small. During my recovery in Styal each person close to me had their own unspoken role and input. My main pillar was Paris, who knows me better than anyone, but it was ultimately down to me to get myself out of the dark wood. Mental recovery is not a short process – you have to work at it every day and it can take years to find your normal after a nervous breakdown, and yet it can take so little time to slide into old behaviour and poor mental health if you're not careful.

Communication is also vital. If I don't speak to Paris about what I'm feeling and thinking, we're not going to have a lasting marriage. Simple as that. Unlike my grandmother, Paris is not a mind reader. Let's face it, relationships are built on talking honestly with each other. If I'm not listening to my coach's input then that relationship is not going to work. Part of the skill of communication is not just about sharing, it's also about listening to the other person's view without interrupting them, and letting them be heard. You need to communicate honestly and regularly with your support team if they are to be good cornermen or women who can help you in your fight. As a boxer, I'm always open to developing and learning something new, and listening helps me be a better dad and husband.

Step Four: Nature

Back in Morecambe from 2015–2017, in the haze of alcohol and drugs, broken sleep and paranoia, I didn't know what normal meant any more. But when I was in Styal, just by going back to basics, back to my roots where I'd grown up, I began to feel more like myself again. And there were no temptations. We'd go walking with the dogs in the woods, chat about stuff, and enjoy silence. Nature is something we should all be made to immerse ourselves in every day of our lives as it has an amazing calming effect. You sit on a beach and watch the waves crashing, the way they have done for millions of years, and you can find peace; your breathing slows and your heart stops beating so fast. By noticing the small miracles around you, it's as if your body blows a sigh of relief. I don't believe that humans belong inside. We are at our happiest when we're connected to the natural elements, and that's been true for hundreds of thousands of years. These days, I love nothing more than riding down Morecambe seafront on my bike early in the morning, singing into the wind as I whizz past the smiling statue of Eric Morecambe. I like the big sky and the distant mountains of the Lake District to the north; nature charges my soul up.

With bipolar disorder, your mood can change twenty times in an hour. But when I'm in nature my moods don't jump about in such a volatile way. When I was in Styal, after a few walks in the forest, with the dogs, my dad and brothers constantly keeping me active, I began to feel a bit different, as if perhaps the internal storm clouds were shifting and the sun was peeking through. The therapist I still went to see each Friday said my time in nature and returning to where I came from was helping to improve my mental health.

Step Five: Sleep

The next improvement while we were in Styal was I started getting much more sleep. There's a couple of reasons to explain this: fresh air makes you tired, and nature gets you in sync with yourself; and I was having big helpings of both. Also, I wasn't as stressed as before, since I'd taken away the negative antagonists, so come the evening my mind was less anxious.

The ideal amount of sleep for adults is eight hours, and it's eleven hours for kids. The land of nod is vital to us as human beings; it not only recharges our brain cells and helps improve our mood, it also keeps our hearts healthy, strengthens mental wellbeing, reduces cortisol – the stress chemical – in our bodies, helps absorb new things into our memory, as well as improving concentration. Sleep deprivation for someone with poor mental health is bad news, particularly those with bipolar disorder, as it can trigger manic behaviour. It also weakens your immune system. To ensure a good night's sleep it's best not to eat a few hours before bed, nor to exercise, or look at a tablet or smartphone, or drink coffee. And as for alcohol, while it can knock you out, the quality of the sleep you have after a few drinks is patchy and unfulfilling.

Another win from a good night's sleep is you wake up earlier, and if you can get in the habit of getting up with the light, you put your own mark on the day rather than hitting the *doze* button and going back to bed. With the latter, the day owns you, and you feel you're letting yourself down. It only takes a thought like *I'm lazy, I never get up*, to start your day on the wrong track. These days I pop out of bed and go straight for a jog before my mind even knows what's happening. I've formed that habit and so can you.

By following a simple routine of gentle early starts, walks in the woods and sunny people surrounding me, I started to feel like myself. I had begun to form a routine, and that routine felt like safety; scaffolding that was holding me up. You need predictability in your life when you're struggling with mental health.

Hopefully, so long as I live by my main medicine – that is to say, a positive environment and routine, plenty of sleep, exercise and lots of it, a sense of purpose and light and love around me – I will keep the demons at bay.

Dip Mode: It's OK When You Slip

You might think that, having written these steps, I have it all worked out. I don't. A coda to this story is that when I finally returned to Morecambe after six months of living peacefully in Styal, I soon became depressed again. I started falling into old habits and hanging out with the wrong people. But to be fair, they didn't make me drink. I did. I did it all myself. Every person is responsible for their own fall in life. It's vital you accept the consequences of your behaviour and take ownership of your actions going forward so you can start to respect yourself again.

Looking back, I wouldn't change one thing in my story, even if you offered to remove the tragic chapters. In my opinion everything happens for a reason, everything goes the way it's supposed to go, and I am where I'm supposed to be. I'm a much better person than I was before my breakdown. I had relapses along the way. I suspect there is a lot more pain in my story and a lot more pain in the way I fight. But I feel like I have a lot more compassion for others and I'm gentler now (at least out of the ring!).

So, for a time I dropped from grace and fell briefly back into 'dip mode' (my code phrase for when the black dog has my soul in its jaws). But it wasn't to last for long. When you're in recovery you need to cut yourself some serious slack; these aren't flabby dossers you're up against, they're Minotaurs and Hydras. You're almost certainly going to slip on your journey back to health and maybe get gored or poisoned, but what you must tell yourself is that it's OK and that you've not gone back to square one. Don't fall out with yourself. Be your own best coach and tell yourself that tomorrow you'll be back on track.

RE-TRAIN YOUR MIND & MENTAL HEALTH

FURIOUS WORKOUT VI

Good morning, warrior. You're looking handsome and beautiful today!

1 Minute 30 Second Warm-up

- Jog on the spot for 20 sec
- Bounce on the spot for 20 sec
- Swivel hips for 20 sec, then the opposite way
- Kick legs out and shake for 10 sec

10 Minute Fast Session
(Remember: hydrate and rest for 30 sec after each)

- Sprint on the spot for 30 sec
- Walking lunges x 15
- Jump squats x 15
- Press-ups x 15
- Sit-ups x 15
- Bicycle sit-ups x 15
- Half sit-ups/stomach crunches x 15
- Squats x 10
- Leg lunges x 10
- Freestyle shadowboxing for 1 minute: bouncing around on the balls of your feet, and moving around the room, pretend you are in a boxing ring and throw different combinations of punches

Warm-down
- Sit on floor, legs straight out, touch toes
- On floor, one leg straight, one leg in, touch toes for 10 sec, then switch leg
- On floor, back straight, feet back and pressed together, push thighs down for 10 sec
- Standing up, pull one knee up, holding foot with hand, feel burn in thigh, switch leg
- Rotate hips for 30 sec then switch in other direction

It's simple: our body is ruled by our mind. It dictates our happiness, the way we perceive others, our fear levels . . . everything. In this chapter we're going to start by focusing on how the brain is made up and why it's important to know what it does right, and what it gets wrong. As sophisticated as we seem as human beings, we'll learn that we're two-thirds animal instinct, which explains a lot in my case! We're also going to discover how to flip our mindset and mood from negative to positive, how to be our own best coach – partly by removing negative triggers and people from our day – and finally how to practise gratitude in order to bring good things into our lives.

Three Brains For the Price of One

Strap yourself in for this amazing bit of science, fellow space cadets. According to some very intelligent person, anything between 70,000 and 100,000 thoughts scramble, scream and sneak their way through our brains each and every day. I never knew I was so thoughtful!

What we *feel* is a result of what our brain has *told* us to feel, but it's important to know that the brain is often on autopilot. There's more than a grain of truth when someone sarcastically says, 'Has your brain disengaged?'

The more familiar you are with doing a task, the more automatic your actions become, because the brain, thinking it's got everything covered, takes a mental break and goes off for a holiday in Marbella or wherever it is brains like to take a vacation. But this reflects our daily lived experience and explains how we can set off in the car, arrive an hour later somewhere and ask ourselves how in the hell we got there, with no recollection of the journey whatsoever.

Although it's an amazing instrument and has achieved extraordinary things in mankind's relatively short history, our brain is actually quite lazy when it comes to cross-checking information and scenarios. If it finds itself in a situation that it has not encountered before, it digs about in our internal hard drive and pulls out a response based on something similar that happened to us in the past. *Or* our brain panics because it's a situation alien and unknown to us, and so it sends us off into our ancestral fight or flight behaviour just to be safe and sound. This can place us unnecessarily on our guard and make us anxious, as if there really is something bad coming to get us, when often there isn't. It's just our brain being over cautious.

Here's another example of our brain running in cruise control. Have you ever met someone you took an instant dislike to, or conversely found yourself smiling at a stranger like they were your new best mate? This is called the 'halo and horns effect', which was first written about by the American psychologist Edward Thorndike a hundred years ago. This phenomenon happens because rather than go to the trouble of getting to know someone, our grey matter tells us how to feel, because unconsciously this awful or perfect stranger reminds us of someone we've once known and either loathed or liked, and who is stored in our memory. When you find yourself smiling at the traffic warden as he or she gives you a ticket, they're probably reminding you of someone you knew!

To counter these 'automatic' behaviours, try to start watching yourself like you're in a cinema and you're on the screen: take some time out and observe and listen to yourself. What you'll see or hear are repetitive trains of thought, or old opinions and self-criticisms that are now redundant and need refreshing, like an update on a smartphone. If your brain is recycling old thoughts, which then create old negative feelings, then you're going to end up living in a cycle of historic negative emotions. The better you get at observing yourself and the skin you're in, the quicker you'll get to work out what makes you tick.

So if we agree that our brain is unreliable and that our thoughts are rarely 100 per cent accurate, it's not too much of a stretch to think that we can filter our thoughts and change the messages we are sending to ourselves. We're not exactly the finished article. Well, I'm certainly not, and according to people smarter than me our brains are still evolving. In the 1960s, Paul MacLean, an American neuroscientist, came up with a theory that divided the brain into three regions, each one with a different job description. Newer theories have emerged, but MacLean's take on the brain is an easy-to-understand description of the different impulses that drive us in our heads.

- **1. The lizard brain (or the basal ganglia)** is the primal part of your brain where your instinctive behaviours spring from. It's also known as the Reptilian complex, and gets its name because it used to be believed that the brains of reptiles and birds were dominated by these motivations. The lizard part of your brain controls your breathing and heart rate, your fear, hunger and anxiety, as well as your sensation of pain, touch, smell, thirst and sexual urges. It even tells you when to sleep and when to wake. The lizard brain deals with the most primitive aspects of being human: it is responsible for keeping you alive. If it sees fit, it will take charge of the rest of the instincts in your brain and shut them down temporarily to ensure survival. This is why seemingly normal people who find themselves backed into a stressful situation can sometimes transform into fierce warriors, or turn and run on legs that they never knew could go so quick.

- **2. The horse brain (or the limbic system)** is the emotional centre of our brain and is where our urge to care for others and be cared for comes from. It gets the name because neuroscientists first believed that animals that share these brain traits include horses, dogs and cats. The horse brain governs the emotions of love, hate, jealousy, pride and happiness. It's where we store old and new memories, which are used to guide us in how we act in certain social situations, or how we respond emotionally to different experiences and even smells. It's also where motivation and purpose live, which is why when we are emotionally invested in something we put all of our efforts into that challenge.

- **3. The human primate brain (or the neocortex)** is the home in our brains for rational thought, creativity and imagination. This is the most recently evolved part of our brains. It is found in other primates too, but for them is smaller and less developed. Our neocortex is likely to be responsible for why the human race has dominated all other species on the planet. It also allows us to try and reason with our natural impulses.

With all the thoughts and signals racing through our minds at any one time, these 'three' brains have to decide the right reaction for each of us in a fraction of a second. No wonder our brains cut corners to save time. But it's this corner-cutting that we can use to our advantage.

People who suffer from depression produce less dopamine, which reduces the stress chemical we produce called cortisol. When we exercise we feel better because it lowers cortisol levels and forces us to create dopamine, which not only helps us to be more alert and engaged, but allows us to be happier. When we smile we release yet more dopamine. Now, the three amigos between our ears are about as alert to fake smiles as one of my vanquished opponents is to one of my feints. The upshot is that our brain responds to our smiles whether they're genuine or not; it doesn't bother checking for witnesses. This is the good bit, stay with me!

When you smile, a series of muscles and nerve endings in your cheeks come together and signal to the brain that you're happy. Transmitters in your brain then produce a hit of dopamine so that you continue to feel like this. So, if you feel fed up and stressed, make yourself smile – you'll feel like a nutter but keep doing it anyway. Your brain doesn't know the difference and sends the dopamine anyway. In other words, it's possible to trick ourselves into feeling better. And before we know it we *do* feel better. And from this positive place we can continue making positive changes.

No doubt you've all heard of mindfulness, which is the practice of learning to be more aware of your thought processes, so that you can consciously decide not to entertain thoughts that will upset or harm you. A good analogy someone once told me is to imagine that you are being towed behind a boat on waterskis. The boat is your brain and the rope is your thoughts. If you're being taken some place mentally that makes you feel bad or unhappy, then all you have to do is let go of that bleeding rope and make yourself think of something else. And you'll protect yourself from further mental harm. But when it comes to me personally, I have a few particular self-preservation techniques that help me in my fight against the blue corner . . .

The Whoop-Whoop Effect

Whenever my mood starts to dip and I catch my thoughts telling me bad stuff, I do the same thing. Just as I feel my energy dropping, I muster as much strength as I can to break through the lead overcoat of depression forming and I jump about shouting 'whoop-whoop'. I 'whoop-whoop' five times, as if my life depends on it. Just by doing this, I am changing my mood and distracting my mind from its current negative trail of thought. Before I know it, I'm in a happier mood. Try it. If you can say 'whoop-whoop' five times very loudly without smiling, I'll give you a medal.

If I find myself dipping emotionally, I also try to identify the irrational thinking behind it and instead concentrate on positive things. When I look back on my life and the times when nothing seemed to be going right for me, I think a large part of this was probably because I kept saying to myself, 'Nothing ever goes well for me. I'm always going to be unlucky.'

I genuinely believe that what we focus on becomes real. When I had a mental breakdown, one bad thing seemed to happen to me after another. Ten days after my Klitschko win, the IBF stripped me of my title because I wasn't able to negotiate a date against mandatory contender Vyacheslav Glazkov, because of a rematch clause with Klitschko. I then broke my ankle in training in Holland and had to postpone that fight. If you allow your thoughts to be washed along into the negative pool, things have a habit of getting worse and worse.

However, you can change that cycle. The morning after Halloween 2017, I said to my wife: 'Monday morning, Paris. I'm on a mission to become the heavyweight champ again.' I was the man who'd cried wolf a thousand times, always making empty promises that I was ready for a comeback, but this time I felt different. I believed it. The positive wheels were turning. The very next day I called Ben Davison to see if he would train me. Then I went for my first run in ages. I was actually too fat to run (28 stone), so I walked instead, and while looking at Instagram on my phone I saw Deontay Wilder's post: a picture of me, extremely obese and bent right out of shape, white as a sheet. It read: 'Even if I had fought him in his prime I would have knocked him out. He's finished and he'll never come back.'

That was the spur I needed. My positive surge was back, and it would not be broken this time. 'Everything is going to be OK,' I told everybody. The response was, 'Why even bother training? You'll never get back in the professional ring.' Despite this, by thinking positively and with God's intervention, I got my boxing licence back and was signed off as sane and well by the doctor who'd cautioned my dad that I was probably going to take my own life. I believe that good things happen when we look for the sunshine.*

. . .

A Healthy Body = a Healthy Mind

As I've said, I keep most of my demons at bay these days by exercising multiple times during the day. On Sundays I give my body a much-needed rest but start feeling low because my body is not enjoying the usual level of endorphins and dopamine produced as a result of cardio work (I like to run or cycle), weights, sparring and pad work. On this day, I try to be *even* more aware of what my thinking is up to, checking the negative thoughts I'm having and trying to be a kind coach to myself.

From Monday to Saturday I start my day with exercise

---

* If you are experiencing depressive or suicidal thoughts, please seek professional help immediately. Everyone's mental health is different and responds to different treatments. Focusing on positive thoughts does not work for everyone.

because I know the mental pay-off is immediate and it starts my motor in a positive way. Just knowing that I've done something good for myself makes me feel mentally stronger, and like I'm ready to deal with what the day will throw at me.

In order to get myself into the right frame of mind to get out of bed in the first place to exercise, I've had to re-programme my thinking. Remember, our natural tendency is to needlessly worry and catastrophise; this isn't and our fault, it's the way we are wired. Humankind has been around for 2.8 million years and for the majority of that time we've evolved under dangerous conditions; as recently as 15,000 years ago we were being hunted by predators. That's why we haven't grown out of these daft extremes of behaviour – we're either crapping ourselves with fear, or we've lost all perspective, seeing the red mist and overreacting to trivial things. It's even harder for people with depression who suffer acute anxiety caused by an increase of cortisol released by the brain.

To think myself into a happy place, my mental routine is that I practise gratitude before my eyes are even open, and it seems to quell the negative thoughts. I thank the Lord for my blessed life, for my family, for the day ahead and all its possibilities. By being grateful for the positive aspects of my life, I find that I can create even more positive things to look forward to. Remember, no matter how dark our life can become at times, there are always slivers of light to hold on to if we choose to look for them. Try this approach below . . .

Three Reasons to be Grateful

As soon as you wake up tomorrow morning, focus on three things that you are grateful for. Write them down here, or on a scrap of paper.

Morning Thanks

1.

2.

3.

Before you go to bed tomorrow evening and start nodding off to sleep, do the same again; thank your god or the universe for three new good things that have happened to you during the day.

Evening Thanks

1.

2.

3.

Gratitude gets easier with practice and I promise you the results are fast. Biologically speaking, you're training your mind into a positive habit and every time you send these positive messages to your brain it releases the 'feel good' chemicals as a reward for your gratitude, quickly lightening your mood.

Box(ing) Breathing

Life coaches and psychologists have long sold the benefits of getting up and easing your way into the day by meditating. Meditation is about relaxing and quieting the mental noise between your ears so you can plug into the stillness. It doesn't require whale music, burning candles, or sitting cross-legged for hours on end to be achieved. These days meditation has become a bit more portable. It can be done before you climb into a boxing ring, onto a bus, or even onto your mother-in-law's sofa!

Try this little 'quick-win' exercise (I highly recommend it for tired parents with short fuses and extremely annoying kids!):

1. With your eyes closed, take a deep breath in through your nose and slowly count to four. You should be able to feel your lungs filling with air.

2. Continue to hold your breath inside as you count to four.
3. Slowly exhale out of your nose for four seconds.
4. And repeat. Try to repeat the first three steps for a few minutes.

This is called 'box breathing', and it can make you feel calmer as the mental noise dies down around you and you focus on your breathing. Studies have shown that this technique may clear the mind, relax the body and even improve your focus, because it feeds oxygen to the brain in a very controlled and calm way.

Beware Negative Dossers

Earlier in the book I talked about a support network and the need to have positive people around you. If you encounter negative people during your day, try to step out of their range and observe them, and the effect they are having, from a distance. You can't really see the negativity until you remove yourself from it. And by removing yourself – which is not possible if you're at work, in a board meeting, or on a sports field – I'm meaning mentally tune out of their negative range. Just by being aware of this, you are separating yourself from them. The longer you allow yourself to be tainted by their negativity, the more you'll absorb it and feel low.

You can't surround yourself with 100 per cent positive strangers once you leave the house; that would be a little weird, like *The Truman Show* or something. And let's face it, it'd be boring after a while if everyone was nice to you all the time! But you *can* make a choice whether you're going to allow yourself to be affected by the person who challenges you to a fight at the traffic lights or rise above it. Negativity breeds negativity. Really, what is the point of getting hit by someone else's idiot stick? If I'm with negative people, within an hour I'll become negative. As soon as I sense bad vibes around me when I'm with my brothers and dad or at home with Paris and the kids, I say: 'Let's be positive. We're able-bodied and well. Let's do something useful today; let's focus on the things we can do. We can walk, we can breathe freely.' Usually the response is a cushion being thrown at me, but I don't mind.

Having been through what I have, I tend to feel sorry for the negative people now. You never know what is going on in somebody's life and why they are acting as they are. They could have been the victim of terrible things, which have ended up shaping their personality. I know from personal experience that if I hold on to grudges I'll only end up attracting more negativity to me, and it soon comes buzzing like a swarm of wasps.

So make sure you cut negative dossers a little slack, and keep curious about the other people you meet in your day. Remember:

Try to never judge a book by its cover – you don't know what someone is like until you've given them the benefit of letting themselves down.

For all that you may think that I talk a lot, I'm also a good listener and I like to hear other people's stories. The more you listen to others, the more you realise we've all got demons we're fighting. Some people are just better at covering them up than others.

Creating Positive Habits and Routine

As I said earlier in the book, the path towards mental equilibrium lies in a positive routine, which can provide a scaffold to support you through the day. For anyone who has bipolar disorder it's especially important to have predictable milestones to balance the manic episodes. It doesn't take long for routine to become habit. My morning routine during the Covid-19 pandemic looked like this:

7.30am: Alarm goes off
8am: Breakfast and industrial amounts of coffee
9am: Morning circuit workout with Paris (one hour)

11am: Go for a four-mile run

1pm: Healthy lunch

2.30pm: Weights, strength work

Early evening: Ten-mile bike ride or five-mile run

Scientists reckon that only about 40 per cent of our actions are consciously made by us; the rest are automatic and habit-based. It's very easy to create bad habits and we do this unconsciously. But if a habit makes you feel good, be it going for a morning walk or listening to a motivational song or podcast, this good habit can quickly become a part of your life. We are only as good as our habits, because it's our habits that inform our actions and identity. So if you're unfit, out of shape, overweight or unhappy, you've likely got bad habits. To really progress in ourselves and our lives I think we need to be more aware of what our habits are, and if they are bad ones we need to root out the damaging behaviours.

You can't be a reformed alcoholic and be hanging out in pubs, or an ex-drug addict still living next to a dealer. To stop a bad habit you have to remove yourself from the environment that feeds it. Replace a bad habit with a good one. Design a routine into which the new habit will fit. We all have good and bad habits. I used to remove tomatoes from my sandwiches and throw them away, but then I developed a habit of ordering them with my food and gradually built up to eating all of them.

Remember: not one of our habits is fixed; each can be remoulded or replaced with a fresh one. There's one condition for this to happen, though – you have to believe you can change your habit to actually do so, and then you have to make the decision to change it.

Triggers

Let's say a person has a habit of going to the pub every day they're at work. They're spending more than they want to and have developed a beer belly. Despite trying to eat a healthy salad at lunch they still find themselves going to the pub with their mates and ordering something to eat and drink.

To get to the root of a bad habit, we first need to ask **how often** is this behaviour happening? In our example, let's say it's at lunchtime at the pub on three days out of five. Next is a harder question. We need to ask **what is the trigger** for going to the pub? Boredom? Hunger? Thirst? You can have positive triggers too. But triggers often relate to things that unbalance our thinking and can make us feel bad about ourselves – and they're often unconscious. Next time you become low in yourself, examine the feeling in your gut and sit with it. Do you feel insecure? Angry? Guilty? Try and pin down if it was something in particular that was said to you that set off a trail of thought that led to an ill feeling inside you. With our pub-goer, perhaps they pass a place each morning that reminds them of a sad memory or person. The more we get used to identifying the triggers that are sending us off down the wrong thought path, the better we'll get at avoiding these negative dead-ends in the future. In many cases, it's quite possible that someone close to us may have said something by accident. I found that when I was trying to get better it was unhelpful to be constantly asked if I was all right as it reminded me of the dark days. It reminded me that something was still wrong with me, and then I would start falling down a muddy slope of depression again. If this is the case, you must communicate to the people in your support network so they know and can stop doing it.

The final part of changing a habit is to figure out what the reward or incentive is that is driving us to this behaviour in the first place. In our pub example, is the person lonely or unhappy on their own – so justifies being there in the company of their friends? Once we're aware of the reward that is driving us, it's much easier to look for a new habit and routine that fulfils that desire. Should our pub-goer be looking to hang out with their friends or family somewhere else? If we realise a reward is destructive or bad for us, we can start to work towards a new reward and a new habit.

I'll leave you with this piece of advice to stew on. If you get stuck in bad ways with your mental health, and if you develop habits or thoughts that you're ashamed of, there is a way back. And forgiveness is part of this. You may need to ask forgiveness of others you've let down with your behaviour. Believe me, I've done my fair share of that. But you also need to forgive yourself. It's a true relief in life. You're carrying a burden with you otherwise. As long as you are dedicated to changing your ways and habits, and you commit to working on your mental health or getting professional support, you're on your way back.

THE POWER OF EXERCISE: FOR BOXING AND LIFE

FURIOUS WORKOUT VII

Top of the morning to you, you beast! Today we're going to do two sets.

2 Minute Warm-up

- Jog on the spot for 20 sec
- Toe touches x 10
- Cross your legs, slowly touch toes for 10 sec x 2
- Bounce on the spot for 20 sec
- Swivel your hips for 20 sec, then the opposite way for 20 sec
- Kick legs out and shake for 10 sec

20 Minute Session

(2 x 10 min sessions. Remember: hydrate and rest for 30 sec after each exercise)

- Jogging on the spot: left straight punch, right straight punch for 1 minute
- Jump squats x 15
- Press-ups x 10
- Sit-ups x 20
- Bicycle sit-ups x 20
- Half sit-ups/stomach crunches x 20
- Squats x 20
- Leg lunges x 15
- Freestyle shadow boxing for 1 minute

1 min break after first set. Then repeat set.

Warm-down

- Sit on floor, legs straight out, touch toes
- On floor, one leg straight, one leg in, touch toes for 10 sec then switch leg
- On floor, back straight, feet back and pressed together, push thighs down for 10 sec
- Standing up, pull one knee up, holding foot with hand, feel burn in thigh, switch leg
- Rotate hips for 30 sec then switch in other direction

For me, health is everything. I think physical activity is the most natural thing on earth to get you mentally in tune with yourself and to boost your wellbeing. Exercise strengthens your heart and reduces stress, it helps your blood circulation and it can even send you to sleep. You only have to look at the rewards it brings to realise that exercise is an evolutionary gift: you feel better on the inside and you look better on the outside. As we've said before, on a chemical level what's happening in the brain when we exercise is that serotonin, endorphins and dopamine, our energy and 'feel-good' chemicals, are released into the body as a reward for your workout. We were born to run, swim and fight, not to be inactive or cooped up. Exercise helps me feel less lacklustre and more pumped up, mentally and physically.

The more we exercise, the less chance there is of the body developing cortisol (the stress hormone that we discussed in the last round), which can make us feel anxious and depressed when its levels are high. Cardio (cardio-vascular) exercise is particularly good at combating cortisol and raising your heartbeat. Your heart is a muscle like any other and it needs to stay fit. A strong heart will deliver more oxygen to cells in your body, which enables your body to burn more fat during exercise and when you rest. It also clears the mind. If I have a problem I'm mulling over, by the time I finish my cardio exercises I've usually solved it. From Monday to Saturday I try to do cardio in the morning and in the evening, and it helps me start and finish my day with a positive mindset.

Rise and Shine!

The early bird becomes heavyweight champion of the world

After exercising, I defy you not to feel a sense of self-satisfaction and wellbeing. That's a big pay-off for just a little bit of cardio! You also respect yourself for doing it and you feel calmer in the world. It's important to build on the happy thinking we talked about in the last round: starting the day with not only positive and grateful thoughts but with physical action; anything that gets a sweat on and makes your heart beat quicker. Exercise, positivity, being in a happy environment and completing goals are my remedy to depression and they have made me a sunnier, more enthusiastic person in all my roles: dad, husband, son and brother.

If you can cycle to work, do yourself a favour and get on your wheels, spin the pedals and get your heart racing. If your commute is runnable, get your pins out and your arms pumping. I appreciate that for many of you, work dictates that you can't exercise as much as I do and with the same flexibility. But what's to stop you getting up an hour earlier and making time for your body? Because it's not just your body that benefits, it's your mind, your outlook on life, and your effect on those around you.

Look around your office first thing in the morning. Who looks like a zombie who's wandered in off a film set, with grey skin and bags under their eyes? And who is bright-eyed and awake, cheeks full of colour, bouncing around like they're on a pogo stick? I'd bet that *The Walking Dead* cast haven't already exercised before sitting down. And they're not going to be set up well for the challenges of the working day either. It's scientifically proven that physical movement keeps our minds sharper. This is because when we exercise we are not only pumping more blood and oxygen to our muscles, but to the brain as well. When we are stressed, stationary or lying down, the brain is starved of this healthy flow, and the crafty cortisol gets in instead.

Studies have found that older people who exercised for an hour three times per week demonstrated heightened cognitive abilities, compared with people who did less exercise or none at all. These superior mental skills included quicker processing of information and better attention, as well as improved time-management skills.

Exercise really does make us sharper mentally and brings out the best in us. Feeling like a sloth can bring you down. When you're out of shape you feel lazy, unmotivated and disconnected from your physical self. Depression's best friend is apathy, that horrible state when you just can't be bothered to do anything that might lift your spirits even though you know you should.

If I go to the gym I feel great; more blood is flowing through my veins and I feel alive. As I mentioned earlier, I love exercising outdoors too. I go to nature reserves to unwind and keep my mindset positive, just as I enjoy running by the sea – the open horizon feels good for my spirit. Sometimes I jog to local ruins, making my way through green fields, alongside stone walls and under huge skies. It doesn't matter if it's raining, it's like it's giving my soul a rinse. I noticed a massive boom in jogging during the pandemic, as if people realised that exercising would help release some of the stress that uncertainty brings, giving them back a feeling of control.

Exercise is a habit I don't ever want to break again, because I know my life literally depends on it. When I stop exercising, part of me starts to die, fading away like a withering plant; it's my sanity and my sunshine. My grandfather on my mum's side trained every day until his last, when he died doing physical work at the age of eighty-five. He inspires me to be the same; I want to be working my body on the day of my last breath too. It's true that nobody likes getting older, for though we might grow a little wiser (here's hoping), feeling our bones stiffen and hearing our joints creak are signs that we're not here for ever and that every day is a footstep towards meeting our Maker. I don't know about you but I want to arrive fit and healthy when I meet St Peter, so if he tells me to stop kidding myself and points me south to the land of fire and brimstone, I can take a long run-up and bounce off a cloud over them Pearly Gates!

If you can get dressed, feed yourself and move freely, you have more to be grateful for than you will probably ever realise. Often, it's only once something is gone that we realise its value and how much we miss it. Exercise is free, the medicine with no side effects, the mental balm that calms the white noise and gives you moments of pure existence rooted in the present. Your mind stops thinking of tomorrow or yesterday and just lets you be.

· · ·

I mentioned earlier my pal Shaun Gash, who lost the ability to walk twenty years ago. He works out like a demon: 500 sit-ups, 100 bench presses; to him that's nothing. He goes for five-mile rolls on the beach, raises money for charities and runs the basketball league he started. Nothing stops that man. Unless you're unable to move your body, or if your mental problems require professional help to get you off the couch (and if that's the case you should seek help), there's really no excuse for not exercising.

Regular exercise is proven to:

- Boost energy
- Increase motor function
- Improve quality of sleep
- Enhance self-esteem
- Fight depression
- Boost sex drive
- Aid digestion
- Strengthen the immune system
- Fight addiction and cravings like sugar because it provides you with dopamine, the 'reward' chemical
- Help with the symptoms of Parkinson's disease
- Fight Alzheimer's

It can also reduce the likelihood of developing:

- Heart disease and stroke
- Type 2 diabetes
- Colon cancer and breast cancer

- Premature death
- Osteoarthritis
- Other forms of dementia

That's quite a persuasive list!

If you still need convincing, in an experiment that followed two groups – one was runners and the other didn't exercise at all – the runners, it concluded, lived an average of three years longer, enjoying a better quality of life as a result of improved health. Or, to put it another way, scientists reckon that for every hour spent running we roughly add another seven hours to our life. Am I convincing you to start?

If you've had a break from exercise for whatever reason, there's no time like the present to get back into it, and there are so many different ways to get fit. Whatever you do, choose something that you *enjoy*; yes, it should be tiring if you're to get the real benefits from it, but it shouldn't feel like punishment and something you dread. If your body doesn't enjoy it, it will be more of an effort to embed it as a part of your routine. So, if you're starting from scratch, remember me when I took my first run at 28 stone. I lasted no more than a few metres before my body went on red alert and told me it was dangerous to push myself after months of self-neglect. So I walked, and that was where I started my campaign to come back and do what I did. Be your body's coach, not a hard-arse sergeant major. The better your talk to yourself, and the more encouraging and self-motivating you are, the further you'll go.

Take running as an example. We all have different levels of fitness and if you're not a natural runner then take it slowly, gradually building up your mileage. But likewise, if it's your first time and you never ran at school or when you were growing up, you may be pleasantly surprised to find that you're better than you think. Often the hardest stride to take is the first one. And once you take the next few strides and build up some momentum, much of the mental battle – often the hardest bit – is over. Some of you reading this will be seasoned athletes and know your body well. For others, if you've been out of the 'ring' for a while when it comes to exercise, perhaps be aware of the time that's elapsed since you were last in shape. Respect your body and don't dive straight into a beasting half-marathon. There are no medals for overdoing it. This leads to a larger point. Even if you are fit or get into tip-top condition, don't push it too hard. Some fighters leave all their energy and fitness in the gym, and when it comes to the moment to fight, when they need to be at their peak, they're sapped of energy because they have over-trained. I'd rather be healthy and a little unfit than over-trained. At least when you're a little unfit, you're out of breath but you can recover and go back at it again. When you're over-trained from too much rigorous exercise you can get stuck in one gear, where you haven't got enough snap. This makes it hard to do anything about it when it comes to a moment where you need to perform or be at your best. It's like being under water.

My Training Camp Routine

Every training camp I enter in preparation for a fight is different. I may need to employ a different strategy or even be at a different weight depending on the fighter I'm facing. I often bring in different trainers to work on my weaknesses as we can always improve. During those parts of my career when I was unwell, my training camps would mostly be weight-loss camps, as I was ballooning up in weight between fights. But I'm proud to say that since my comeback I've been staying fit and at a good weight between fights, so I can concentrate on sharpening my boxing skills and strategy in the camp, and getting fight-ready, as opposed to feeling like I'm in an extreme Weight Watchers boot camp. I always try to improve and work on different strengths to prepare me for fight night. I can't share all my secrets here (just in case Wilder and AJ are reading!) but here is a breakdown of some of the exercises I did in the run-up to the most recent Wilder fight:

Morning Session

Jump rope

I may look a bit silly doing it, being as big as I am and particularly when I'm only wearing a training shirt and some boxers in the gym, but I love skipping. I use it to keep my footwork fast, and I try lots of different footwork combinations. Skipping is great for warming up, relaxing and for loosening your limbs. It's excellent cardio and I usually do it for about ten minutes.

Shadow boxing

Whether I'm out on the seafront in Morecambe after a run, or in the gym under my trainer SugarHill's watchful eye, shadow boxing is a quality way to develop muscle memory for the ring, and it's also a bloody good workout. You focus on your technique, your combinations and crucially your movement. But you can also improve your speed, power and overall strength and endurance.

Sparring

I'm not afraid to assemble the best fighters in the world to spar rounds with in the build-up to my fights. Wladimir Klitschko, AJ, Daniel Dubois, Joe Joyce . . . I've sparred them all, although I like to keep what goes on in sparring – in sparring. The reason boxers spar is the same as why footballers play friendlies or practice matches: it's the best way to replicate what it's going to be like on fight night in the ring. Of course, you don't get the atmosphere of a real fight, but without enough sparring, a boxer has lost before he or she gets into the ring. You get punch-fit and your body gets used to absorbing pain and processing adrenaline rather than releasing too much cortisol, which is what can happen with time out of the ring. I can go twenty rounds of sparring in a row, which for a big guy like me isn't bad. And preparing for more than twelve rounds makes the fight easier on the night. It gives you confidence that you can go deep into the hurt locker if you're trained for it. Whether you're a boxer or a cyclist or a swimmer or a runner, if you train hard, you'll find it easy when it comes to game night. Towards the end of a camp I begin to wind down the number of rounds I'm doing in readiness for the big night; fewer rounds but sharper skills.

Afternoon Session

More Sparring

Sparring can burn 800 calories an hour. It's great for your sharpness in boxing and your overall fitness. But like I said earlier in this round, beware of over-training. The greatest risk that sparring poses to a boxer is injury: remember, you assemble some of the best boxers to fight you, and deep down they all want to be where you are. When you get into a spar you are putting it on the line. So you have to be mindful to spar enough to get in shape for the fight, but not too much to risk missing the fight though injury.

Bag Work

There are many kinds of heavy bags; they come in lots of different weights and shapes. For uppercuts, under-hooks and overhand punches I'll use angled bags. For a variety of strikes, teardrop and wrecking-ball bags are useful all-rounders. Finally, the standard heavy bag is my best friend for practising concussive punches. For Wilder II, I worked on a 350-pound heavy bag to focus on my strength and power, and to practise my balance, co-ordination and sequences of punches (including eye contact when

I'm throwing these combinations). I'd typically alternate between a round of speed punches (soft) standing square on to the bag, then a round of punch combos (hard), doing six rounds of each, but sometimes I'll do as many as twenty rounds.

Bag work is great for relieving stress if you imagine the bag is your opponent! Typical punching on a heavy bag burns about half the calories of sparring per hour. I don't use a speedball as I don't really think you get much from it other than looking a bit fancy, but I use smaller bags when I want to practise my hand speed and reaction times.

Mitt Work

Choreographed mitt work with my trainer is a good halfway house between sparring and hitting a bag. You agree in advance the combinations you are going to throw, and together you can control the pace. Great fighters and trainers who have been together a long time make mitt work look almost exactly like fighting, because they're so in tune with each other.

Battle Ropes

To work my legs, chest, back and core, I've trained with battle ropes in the past, although I didn't use them for the second Wilder fight. Holding each end of the rope an arm's width apart, you should clench your stomach muscles, squat and keep your back straight and then begin waving the ropes up and down. I'll keep doing this for a few minutes, and then switch things up and do a different set. Waving the ropes side to side works out your core and hips more, whereas moving the ropes in circles works out your shoulders.

Late Afternoon Session

Footwork

Footwork is crucial in boxing for getting yourself in the optimal position to strike your opponent, to switch stance, to elude punches and for cutting off the ring to make sure your opponent has nowhere to run. Most heavyweights are quite flat-footed but I've always prided myself on my ability to dance on the balls of my feet even though I'm as big as I am. I concentrate a lot on my long legs to make them as strong as possible, so that I can move around the ring as fast as possible. We'll do lots of squats, hops on the spot and from side to side, and other footwork exercises like back-pedalling, pivoting and 'Ali shuffling' to make sure I'm as strong and agile as possible. Made famous by Muhammad Ali, the Ali shuffle is simple but tiring if you do it for a while. Keeping your weight on the balls of your feet, switch your legs front and back, keeping your feet facing forward. Skipping is also a good way of refining your footwork, as is shadow boxing.

Weightlifting

I'll lift heavier weights further out from a fight, and then as the bout gets nearer I'll start doing lighter weights to build up my explosiveness. I do a full range of weight training including bench presses, deadlifts, bicep curls, squats, floor lifts, kettle bells and medicine balls. Much of the focus will be on lower body strength to make my legs rock solid so my footwork will be on point. I'll keep the upper body training light as I approach a fight, as recovery is key to strength, and my upper body will already be well conditioned from all my punching. I typically deadlift very heavy weights, from about 210 kilos to as much as 250 kilos, but I don't advise you to do the same.

Bodyweight Training

Alongside weights I'll do a variety of press-ups, clapping press-ups (where you clap between press-ups), tricep dips, chin-ups and planks (forty-five seconds on, ten seconds off, eight sets).

Cardio

As I've said before, I look forward to my training; it's part of my life, part of my routine. The boxing, the running, the strength work, it all rolls into a lovely big 'thank you very much' every day. When I'm preparing for a fight, I'll often do hill running, to test both my mental and physical strength. Whether it's six miles up a mountain in the US, or up a ramp off Morecambe Bay, it's the same: when I'm doing sprints uphill it works on my explosiveness, the longer runs work on my endurance. Ultimately, knowing that I'm climbing that hill or mountain gives me a big mental edge when I know I'm getting close to reaching my peak fitness. I also enjoy cycling, both on the road and on the bike in the gym, rowing in the gym and using the elliptical – all your standard workout machines and equipment.

Recovery Massage

After a tough session, a massage helps to keep me loose and flush out all my stress and anxieties. It's also a time for me to banter with my team as we let off steam after we've done the hard work.

Evening

Three-mile recovery run

To keep my body ticking over, I'll finish the day with a short run so I don't seize up the next day.

Exercise Breakdown

Breaking down what I do to its basics, my main training to get fit as a fighter consists of roadwork (running and cycling), pad work, sparring, weights and aerobic conditioning. Breaking this down even more, there are three kinds of exercise: **aerobic** (aka conditioning or cardio), **flexibility** and **anaerobic.**

Aerobic exercise requires oxygen in your blood, heart and lungs to fuel your body for activities like running or cycling. This is cardio exercise, as we've explored in this round already. When you're unfit you can't get up a flight of stairs without losing your breath, but the fitter you get, the more effectively your body can manage your oxygen intake without getting knackered. Cardio exercise is great for boosting mood, burning calories, getting a good night's sleep, speeding up your metabolism and managing diseases like Parkinson's and dementia. As you build up your stamina, let your exercise regime reflect that by increasing it by a few minutes for each session, and if you're walking, hiking, cycling or running, turn up the pace a bit too.

You'll notice in my Instagram posts with Paris (and the occasional uninvited pint-sized disruptors) that we used a three-tier approach to our cardio workouts: the warm-up, the session itself and the warm-down. The benefit of warming up is it gently gets the blood flowing around your body to all your muscles, and gradually gets your heart pumping faster. During the session itself, it's vital to hydrate regularly if you're not going to fry your brain with dehydration. And then after the session we warm down, stretching off quadriceps (upper thigh muscles), calf muscles, lower back and shoulders.

My Instagram workouts are what you call 'medium intensity interval training', taking short breaks of around thirty seconds between each individual exercise in your cardio session. It's one of three levels of cardio exercise:

- **HIIT (high intensity interval training)** This takes less time but you're going at it full tilt and twice as hard as **MIIT**. Workout time is around 12–15 min. Possible exercises: sprints, speed boxing, spinning, battle ropes.

- **Medium-intensity intervals** Workout time around 15–30 min. Taking as long as required (but not too long, dosser!) to recover between sets of kettlebells, skipping, quick jogging, battle ropes etc. You should still be pushing yourself, just not to the max.
- **Steady-state cardio** Workout time 30–60 min. Keeping at a steady pace so your heart rate is somewhere between 120–150 beats per minute. Includes anything like cycling, jogging and swimming.

The next type of exercise is called **flexibility training**, which aims to minimise the risk of injury by increasing the mobility of the joints. We also use some of these exercises in the warm-down. Tai chi, Pilates and yoga fall under this umbrella. I don't personally do much tai chi, but you will see me doing yoga stretches in particular. Stretching your hips, back, arms and legs is crucial work and will lengthen your muscles and improve how flexible you are. If you have tight hamstrings or tight shoulders, you'll be amazed at how quickly you can change how your body feels, and how much more flexible you can become by doing regular yoga. This work will often strengthen your core in the process as an added benefit.

Finally, **anaerobic** or strength training (also called resistance training) refers to the use of weights to build and maintain muscle. As I outlined in my fight camp workout above, it's always good to balance how much strength training you do, and with your overall fitness target in mind. If you are a long-distance runner, it won't make a lot of sense to put on loads of muscle as that bulk will slow you down.

For a balanced approach with strengthening exercises you should try and work all the major muscles (legs, hips, back, abdomen, chest, shoulders and arms) at least twice a week using weights, press-ups, yoga and Pilates.

It's best to vary all three types of exercises (aerobic, flexibility and anaerobic) so you're not overdeveloping certain aspects of your body. On average, most of my training, across fight camps and when I'm at home, consists of strength and conditioning, running and boxing.

As I've said before, I train from Monday to Saturday. I'm blue on a Sunday as that's the one day I'm not exercising, but I need to give my body a well-earned rest. When you're training your muscles, fibres pull against each other, which is why your muscles can hurt after your workout. When your muscle fibres tear, they do repair themselves so that they grow back stronger and thicker. But recovery is important in this process, otherwise your muscles won't repair themselves properly.

You can't push yourself too hard as you'll cause yourself injury, so listen to your body. There's a difference between being lazy and recognising when your body needs a rest. Your body can self-heal. It's a very smart natural machine, and it will always tell you when it's time for a break.

When Should We Hang Up Our Gloves With Exercise?

In my opinion, never. The Spartans of fifth-century Greece insisted that every citizen be fit for battle until the age of sixty. That should teach us a thing or two about thinking it's all over after fifty. My dad is fifty-three, fit as a fiddle, and the heavy bag in the gym groans when it sees him putting on a pair of mitts to come and give it some punishment. There is no age limit to exercise. If you're a person who has exercised all your life you should try to never stop. It's always harder to return to after a break, but after your first contact with it again it's as easy as pie. It's all relative too. Designing what you do to suit your age and ability is key to not giving yourself an injury. For instance, given that speed walking and jogging are high impact on the joints, as you get older you could vary these exercises with more low-impact sports such as cycling or weights. Strength work, in particular, is extremely beneficial for old bones; muscles get weaker as we get older, but training counters that. Start slowly with weights and steadily progress in repetitions and weight.

Ultimately, it's up to us whether we decide we're old before our time. In China there are outdoor gymnasiums in many public parks, designed to keep pensioners fit. They have monkey bars, stretching machines, bars for leg pull-ups and all sorts. Because they work out every day as part of their routine, Chinese pensioners are able to keep exercising much later into old age – use it or lose it! But let's leave the final word to the Spartans. Before I enter the ring for my fights, I chant 'WE ARE SPARTANS!' with my team. It gets me buzzing. Someone once told me a Spartan story. Philip II of Macedon had been conquering Greece with crushing victories. The Spartans were weak at the time, and legend has it that Philip sent a message to them along the lines of: 'If I invade your land, you will be totally destroyed.' The Spartans replied with one word: 'If.' Philip never dared to attack the Spartans. Their discipline, their bravery, and their mental strength were too strong to be reckoned with. And I take belief and strength from them when I'm wavering.

Behind Every World Champ is a Brilliant Team

You're probably sensing a theme now in this book – you don't have to do it all alone. When it comes down to exercise, ultimately I am the one who has to get up and do some exercise each morning or head to training. And that will be the case with you, too – at the end of the day, you are responsible for your health. But you can draw on the support and team spirit of others.

I am very grateful that for a number of years now I have had a brilliant strength and conditioning coach, Kristian Blacklock, who I met at the start of the training camp for Klitschko back in 2015. I've kept with him ever since. Old Baldy Head (we call each other this) is – along with my brothers – the only remaining member of the original Team Fury. His gym in Ormskirk, Lancashire, is state of the art, and has a great buzz about the place. I'm treated just like anyone else, and my brothers and I regularly train there. There's even a giant mural of yours truly landing a slick right on Deontay Wilder's mush.

I've recently bought a gym in Morecambe to serve as the HQ of the Tyson Fury Foundation (we'll come to why I set up the foundation at the end of the book). I've been training in my gym as I've been writing this book and it's terrific. On the wall is another cracking mural – the Gypsy King throwing yet another pulverising shot at the Bronze Bomber during Wilder II. The only colour in the mural's otherwise monochrome scheme is the emerald green of my gloves.

To be honest, I'm not really bothered about having too many different kinds of machines and bags in my gym. A good boxer trusts in the basics. My favourite Rocky film is *Rocky IV* because, for all the technical equipment Rocky's enormous Russian opponent Ivan Drago and his team use to build him into a human machine, Rocky just goes back to basics – jogging through snow, doing pull-ups and stomach crunches, and chopping wood. There are essentially three key elements to boxing: pad work, sparring and road work. All that scientific stuff means very little to me. You can have all the flash, hi-tech equipment in the world but if you're not a better fighter than your opponent it won't help you.

I owe Kristian a lot for helping me on my comeback, and for putting together workout plans that prepare me for all my fights. Below is a typical strength and conditioning workout that Old Baldy Head devised for me during my training camp in Vegas for Wilder II. Please do not try this at home, and please do not attempt to lift weights unless you are safe and supervised in a gym (otherwise you risk injury).

OLD BALDY HEAD'S VEGAS WORKOUT FOR WILDER II

Start with a pulse raiser: jog on a treadmill or cycle on an exercise bike for ten minutes.

Follow this up with five minutes of mobilisation exercises, like swinging your arms from left to right, or do some shadow 'jabs' using a resistance band. This should be a gentle start to get the blood flowing and to wake up the heart.

To focus on speed and explosiveness, complete five sets of:

Explosive bench presses (140kg) x 5
Jump squats x 5
Bench presses (140kg) x 5
One arm dumb-bell lifts (25kg) x 5
Pull-ups with 30kg weight belt x 10
Dips with 30kg weight belt x 10
Walking lunges x 10
Clap press-ups x 5

Finish with four minutes of Tabata high-intensity training, which works the body aerobically and anaerobically to simulate the explosive bursts of energy required in the ring. Choose four exercises from the six listed below. You should do each exercise for one minute, broken down into two rounds: twenty seconds on and ten seconds rest.

Squats
Burpees
Sprints
Press-ups
Tap squats
Ali shuffle

Warm down for ten minutes with jogging and stretching.

• • •

As I said at the start of this round, my mental health is directly linked to exercising, and Kristian's helped me with both. I want to finish with three takeaways from Old Baldy Head for a healthy life:

- Have a routine. People with good routines in their life are generally happier and more consistent in what they do.
- Hydrate regularly. Drinking plenty of water on a regular basis might sound absurdly simple but so many people don't do this and as a result it makes them hungry and they eat more. We get the majority of the fluids in our body from food as well as water. When you are dehydrated it triggers a hunger response in your body and you start craving food. Water helps every organ function, as well as cleansing your stomach, improving your skin and energy levels. It's the most important nutrient in our diet.
- Take one day at a time and each day as it comes.

MAKING WEIGHT: FINDING YOUR PERFECT SIZE

FURIOUS WORKOUT VIII

We're on it again, let's go! Time to up the ante. This workout is three sets. Good luck!

2 Minute Warm-up

- Jog on the spot for 20 sec
- Toe touches x 10
- Cross your legs, slowly touch toes for 10 sec x 2
- Bounce on the spot for 20 sec
- Swivel your hips for 20 sec, then the opposite way for 20 sec
- Kick legs out and shake for 10 sec

30 Minute Session

(3 x 10 min workouts. Remember: hydrate and rest for 30 sec after each, x 3 sets)

- Freestyle shadow boxing for 30 seconds
- Jump squats x 10
- Press-ups x 10
- Sit-ups x 10
- Bicycle sit-ups x 10
- Half sit-ups/stomach crunches x 10
- Squats with punches x 10 (normal squat with a punch when you stand up)
- Leg lunges x 10
- Burpees x 10
- Star jumps x 10

1 min break after each set. Then repeat.

Warm-down

- Sit on floor, legs straight out, touch toes
- On floor, one leg straight, one leg in, touch toes for 10 sec then switch leg
- On floor, back straight, feet back and pressed together, push thighs down for 10 sec
- Standing up, pull one knee up holding foot with hand, feel burn in thigh, switch leg
- Rotate hips for 30 sec then switch in other direction

Boxers do the craziest things ahead of fights to make the weight required by their division: starving themselves of fluid, running on a treadmill in a sweat suit, cycling in a sauna . . . anything to hit the target weight. Otherwise, they risk disqualification. Some fighters lose as much as 30 pounds in two days. This can be very dangerous and seriously lowers the body's energy levels. Sweat isn't just water, and although fighters are given twenty-four hours to rehydrate and eat as much as they like before competing, the lost salt and electrolytes from cutting weight put the health of your heart at risk. If you cut too much weight, you're potentially putting your body in jeopardy.

Fortunately, in the heavyweight division you can be as heavy as you like, so it's not about meeting a weight for me. Instead it's about finely calibrating my ideal fighting body. I want to be nimble on my feet without being too light to pack a powerful punch – the heavier you get the more power you load into your fists. For the first Wilder fight, my main goal was coming down from 28 stone and fighting the fat. Unusually, in hindsight I think I actually went too far the other way for that first Wilder fight. I ended up weighing in at 18 stone on the scales before the bout. This was probably too light, and was the average weight I was when I was just starting out in my career. The result was it left me weak and feeling a bit drained. Come the fight I didn't have the powerful energy required to finish Wilder the way I wanted.

For Wilder II it was a much better experience. I kept the weight in check and focused on being lean while also packing on a few more pounds of muscle. I hit the scales at 19½ stone of pure British beef. The added weight gave me the strength I required to manhandle and push him into fatigue. It also turned my fists into fairground mallets. Since that fight I've kept fit and maintained a steady weight. When my next fight is confirmed I won't have to waste valuable time at the training camp losing the weight and can instead concentrate on my fighting skills.

In this round we'll cover the two different diets I used for my fights against Wilder and how they worked for me. The rest of the round will be about you and how to find the right balance between looking ripped and feeling comfortable with yourself. Your perfect weight is dependent on how tall you are, how heavy-boned you are, and what body shape you have. When losing weight you need to know *what* you want to lose. If you set a specific weight target, you've more chance of hitting it than if you're vague and non-specific. But more important than the *what* is being really clear first on asking yourself *why* you want to lose your weight. I don't think losing weight should be all about improving the way you look, but more about having a positive impact on your quality of life. Here's a few prompts for you to think about to establish your *why* (although the specifics will be different obviously for everyone):

I want to lose weight because:

- I'm feeling heavy and tired as a result of being overweight
- I look old and drained before my time
- I can't play with my kids or do exercise with others for long as I get out of puff quickly
- I feel self-conscious in my clothes
- I can't get in to last year's trousers
- There's a history of obesity-related diabetes in my family
- I've lost self-control and respect for myself
- I want to feel healthy again, for myself and for my family and friends
- I want to improve my self-image

Everyone needs a strong *why*, a good reason to lose weight. The clearer your *why* is and the more emotionally committed you are, the easier it is to define a good *what*, and to actually get there. If your *why* is to get fit for your daughter's wedding, then you might set your *what* to lose 2 stone.

But another good question to ask yourself is: 'What does my perfect long-term weight look like?' Everyone has a different answer and vision, so whatever feels good to you as a person is all that counts. Set your goal, then set your stall out and achieve it. Your self-talk has to be clear. You can't say: '*Maybe* I'll do this.' Be firm with yourself, but be honest too. A more dramatic weight loss may be achievable for you in the short term, but it may not be sustainable, or the best for you, in the long term, just as me getting down to 18 stone wasn't ultimately my smartest move.

Body Shapes

To better understand weight loss, let's explore the three basic body types: ectomorph, mesomorph and endomorph. We are all a unique combination of all of them.

- **Ectomorphs** are people who have naturally slim bodies with quick metabolisms, and they often have light bones and narrow shoulders. They can find it hard to put on weight and to add muscle because they burn it off so quickly. To build muscle they typically need less cardio and more intense strength workouts with weights. They are more likely to need to eat at least 3,000 calories a day, with plenty of carbs, protein and fat. They probably also need to train less, to allow the muscle to settle without being quickly burned off with too much exercise. Exercise is mostly recommended three times per week for people with predominantly this body type. Ectomorphs are sometimes advised to use supplements like a protein shake before a workout and afterwards to add muscle, but in the first instance they should try to get protein naturally as part of a balanced healthy diet.

- **Mesomorphs** fall in the middle between ectomorphs and endomorphs. They are typically naturally muscular and medium-boned and have good metabolisms (not as fast as ectomorphs but not as slow as endomorphs). They tend to find it easy to lose and put weight on. They can pack on muscle quickly, and because of their long torsos and shorter limbs they are usually good at explosive sports requiring power and speed. If you're a mesomorph, consider yourself lucky.

- **Endomorphs** have larger bone structures and store fat more easily. They could be described as curvy or stocky and have fuller figures. Fat is stored in the belly, on the hips and thighs. They find it harder to lose weight and easier to put it on. They should aim to avoid eating too many carbs and focus on quality fats and protein. Also, they should eat less regularly. They find it easier to convert fat to muscle rather than lose weight. Endomorphs have a slow metabolism so should avoid sitting down for long periods to combat this. CrossFit, running and high-intensity exercises are the best way for them to lose weight. If you're an endomorph, high five! Like me, you're part of the club.

Usually, people are a mix of two body types or shapes. Identifying which shape you are enables you to choose the right foods and exercise. If I'm an endomorph, I'm going to have to accept the fact that it will be harder to look ripped than if I was a mesomorph like Deontay Wilder, who naturally burns fat off quickly. I used to crave a body that was ripped when I took my top off. As a young lad I was always on the plump side and my weight was up and down like a yo-yo. I really wanted to be in top shape as a boxer but because of my body type I found it hard to look shredded. I remember my dad saying to me: 'It's not in your DNA. You're never going to be built like Schwarzenegger, so forget about that. You're here to do one thing and one thing only. You're a fighting man.'

On first impression, some people write me off as a boxer because I don't have the chiselled torso of a statue, just an ordinary dad's body with cheese packs and love handles to boot. I train multiple times per day and am still a chubby fella! All credit to Anthony Joshua for being in such amazing shape. He's had to work very hard to achieve that physique, but he's also got the right body type to be able to look like that. When he was beaten by Andy Ruiz Jr in their first fight in 2019, most people, looking at the two men facing one another, found it hard to imagine that a small overweight American could defeat such an incredible physique. All I can say is, never judge a book by its cover. Ultimately, I'm not interested in how I look. The most important thing is that I am fit for purpose. I train for my own mental wellbeing, because it makes me happy. And I train to do my job well.

This isn't the first time in this book I've said this, but you're only as good as the company you keep. If you're around people who eat fast food all day, you'll eat the same food, but if you share the company of healthy types this will rub off on you and become second nature. Years ago, if you needed to know something it was harder to ask experts and there were fewer books in the library on the subject. We are lucky enough to have more knowledge in this era than ever before. At the press of a button you can Google 'healthy diets'. Up until I began training for the first Deontay Wilder fight I was drinking nearly twenty to thirty cans of Diet Coke per day. It sounds ridiculous but I loved it. Now I know better! It's up to us to educate ourselves.

Finding the Right Weight is About Being Comfortable in Your Own Skin

Every boxer has an ideal fighting weight, one at which they can operate to their maximum ability at both a cardio and strength levels. As I said earlier, my optimum fight weight was around 18 stone – 18½ stone for much of my career – but now I'm older and in my twilight days as a fighter I find that if I come in heavier, I not only have more firepower but I can also absorb more punishment. It doesn't look great and I'm never going to be asked to take my shirt off for a Davidoff commercial, but I've got an exceptional inner engine and I can fight hard till the bell goes at the end of the twelfth round. Carrying the extra weight doesn't affect me but it affects my opponent, as was the case with Wilder, who I dominated in our second fight by leaning on him in the few clinches we had.

We all have a dream size, an optimal weight on the scales that allows us to be light on our feet, to feel energised and happy. Like I've said, I've got to the age now where I realise that my outward appearance doesn't matter, so long as I can do my job as a boxer properly and be a weight that makes me contented in my own skin. I no longer crave that six pack, as I know it's not a reflection of how hard you punch or your fitness level. It's a body type that makes it look like you've stepped out of the pages of a Marvel comic. But, to be honest, in my time I've knocked out twenty-one boxers with six packs!

Everybody is different; we're all various shapes and sizes. If you're naturally bigger boned it may be a struggle to lose a significant amount of weight, and in the long term it may not be realistic trying to be rake thin. It's subjective of course, but sometimes when people lose lots of weight they even get criticised for their head ending up looking disproportionately large for their body, like a lollipop. This does sound like nonsense to me. Sometimes you can't win with what other people say; try not to listen to them. The most important thing in life is to be happy with who you are on the inside before you start worrying about the outside. The goodness within a person is their true measure, not whether they've managed to get down to a thirty-two-inch waist.

As I mentioned earlier, you couldn't get any more ripped than Deontay Wilder was in our second fight; he looked like an Adonis. Then he fights a big old fat fella like me with a bald head and gets plastered. He might have the six pack but I've got the keg! Like I said earlier, I was lighter when I fought Wilder the first time, and ultimately it was maybe part of why I didn't get the victory. It was a similar thing when I fought Otto Wallin in September 2019 at 18 stone 1 pound; again I came in too light. I trained hard with my team but we never properly accounted for the heat in Las Vegas in the middle of the summer, and the extra weight it would take off. I was weighing half a stone less than I should have been. Remember: if you come in under your natural weight it can deplete your energy, sap your strength and make you feel like you're submerged and walking through water. It's called weight drain. It was fifty degrees when I trained for that Wallin fight and we were training twice a day, six times a week. No matter how much I ate I couldn't put the weight back on. And as you may have seen in that fight (or if you watch clips online), I lacked power against Wallin.

The Keto Diet

I first heard about the keto diet when I went to watch my friend Dereck Chisora fight in November 2017 in Monte Carlo. It was while I was there that another friend of mine, Brendan Lyons, who does my security, told me about it. Since the diet allowed me to eat bacon and eggs, sausages, burgers, Diet Coke and Coke Zero I was immediately interested! I didn't believe it would work but I had a crack at it and dropped down to 25 stone in a matter of weeks. I thought, 'Wow, this is the best diet I've ever tried.' I started training with my then coach Ben Davison at the end of 2017 and thanks to him and the keto diet, and a great training camp in Marbella in early 2018, by the spring of that year I was down to 22½ stone (but we'll get to that training camp in a moment).

The ketogenic diet is a high fat, low protein and low carbohydrate regimen which causes the body to burn fat rather than carbs. Most keto diets are 55–80 per cent fat, 15–30 per cent protein and 5–10 per cent carbs. It typically requires you to remove all but 50 grams of carbs from your daily diet. Pasta, bread, potatoes, milk and sugar are replaced with a high-fat index of foods like avocados, coconuts, seeds and red meats. My tailored diet was made up approximately of 50–55 per cent fat, 30 per cent protein and 15 per cent carbohydrates. When there's only a slight presence of carbohydrates, which are turned into glucose, the liver converts fat into fatty acids or ketones, which replace glucose as a source of energy. This is called ketosis and mimics what happens to your body during starvation. Whereas the 'clean' version of the keto diet involves nutritious whole foods with no processed food, the 'dirty' keto diet, which I was on, is less choosy, doesn't insist on organic food, and allows for a greater variety of food, including potatoes, chocolate, chips, pretzels, cheese, and coffee with cream.

The keto diet is safe for most people, but you shouldn't do it if you have conditions involving your liver, pancreas, thyroid or gall-bladder. Long term, some scientists have also pointed out that it may lead to heart rhythm problems. I should point out that like any diet there are some cons, as well as pros, and it won't be right for everyone, so make sure that you talk to a doctor or a registered dietician if you are considering following a ketogenic diet. For some people the cons can include headaches, constipation, dizziness and a lack of nourishment resulting from avoiding fruit and veg. Sometimes it can also increase stress levels and the feeling of being tired, because of a lack of the protein that would otherwise provide energy for your body. You can also feel nauseous as your body gets used to burning fat stores for fuel instead of carbs. I felt some of these unpleasant side effects when I was on the diet. I was training three times a day at my obese weight, so it's no wonder that during my journey back to health I sometimes felt depleted; it was a bit like I was running on empty. Losing all that weight must have taken its toll on my body and at times it was hard being on the diet, but I do think it was worth it. I felt so good when I had eventually lost all that weight. By June 2018, when I faced Sefer Seferi in my first comeback fight after my lay-off from boxing, I was down to below 20 stone.

The keto diet is not normally recommended for athletes as it can rob you of precious energy. My team and I knew that it would leave me lacking in energy at first, but it was something I had to do, and it proved to be perfect for me losing the pounds. I'm a big believer in sacrifice to achieve my goals. I've sacrificed my life for sporting glory, and it hasn't been easy, given that I've got a sweet tooth and a fat-retaining body type. Losing weight is never a quick fix, it's a lifestyle change. There were times in the past when, ahead of a photo shoot, I'd lose weight by watching what I was eating and then pile the pounds back on as soon as I returned to my regular diet. Back then, I had a constant battle with my weight going up and down, whereas these days I've formed new habits and it's less of a struggle.

Wilder I Preparation

A lot changed for me at my training camp in Marbella in early 2018, which ultimately started my preparation for my fight against Deontay Wilder in December later that year (I would have another training camp much closer to the Wilder fight in the US, but my time in Marbella made everything that I achieved that year possible). It was a great and hugely positive experience for me. I was 25 stone going into the camp. My daily diet made a big difference and for seven weeks during the camp it consisted of:

- Breakfast – bacon, cheese, eggs and mayo, no bread
- Lunch – half a roast chicken with mayo
- Dinner – two burgers with cheese and bacon (no buns) and mayo

Thanks to my keto diet, and weeks of hard exercise in which I trained three times per day with the trusted friends and family who came out to support me, my life was transformed. I was running up and down local mountains, training on the beach and inside the gym. Even at 25 stone I was soon able to run up Marbella's La Concha mountain, which was a six-mile climb. It was brutal at first. But I stuck to my diet and new exercise routine and each person in my team played a part in my recovery and weight loss. Everyone was always ready to go to the gym at 7 a.m. or join me running up the hills at the drop of a hat. That said, there wasn't a day that went by where I didn't want to quit and go home, because that would have been the easiest thing to do. I'd only started running in October 2017 and now I was going on runs of up to ten miles per day. In my quest to lose weight, I typically did morning cardio, afternoon weights and boxing in the evening. Remember, the food you eat is just one part of losing weight – you still need to dedicate yourself to exercise and routine, and you need a positive mindset to keep you on course.

Without a clear goal that gave me a strong sense of purpose, I would never have been able to lose so much weight so quickly. If you are looking to shed pounds, I wouldn't recommend doing what I did. Losing that much weight can be dangerous for your body. My intention now is never to have to lose that amount of weight ever again. Weight plays a big part in my mental health. When I put on a lot of weight it happens in tandem with my mental health deteriorating. I get sucked into a black hole which isn't easy to escape from. Training for me is medicinal and maintaining weight control is vital.

Wilder II Preparation

For Wilder II I had a major shake-up in my team and my general approach – both to training and to my diet. I knew I needed to improve to go to the next level, both in terms of boxing and in my health. As I've mentioned before, on the trainer side I replaced Ben Davison with Javan 'SugarHill' Steward to help me be more aggressive. I very much wanted Ben in the team as my number two but he had his reasons for not coming on board and I respect that. I also contacted George Lockhart, the ex-US Marine turned MMA fighter and now top nutritionist and chef to some of the world's best fighters.

George Lockhart became my nutritionist and I don't know how I ever managed without him. His formula for losing weight is consuming moderate quantities of organic, healthy food throughout the day. George is half-Mexican, half-American and he often incorporates Mexican recipes into the delicious meals he makes for me – he's a brilliant cook. He prepares and cooks all the meals himself. During our training camp in Vegas, he made regular visits to the local farmers' market to stock up on fresh, organic foods. I don't like vegetables much so George manages to hide them well in the meals he makes me. On any given day I am taking on 4,500 calories and given that in forty-five minutes I can burn 1,500 calories, I now eat six times per day. Below is an example of a diet plan George designed and then prepared for me:

George Lockhart's Diet Plan for Wilder II

- **Breakfast:** Greek yoghurt and fruits (lots of berries for antioxidants, which may protect your cells against heart disease, cancer and other diseases). Yoghurt is good for boxers and other athletes because it includes calcium for strong bones, vitamin D, which helps your body absorb the calcium, and it's high in protein. It also includes good bacteria that helps your gut health and digestion.
- **Pre-workout shake:** 4,000 milligrams of beta-alanine, a naturally occurring amino acid, which can help build muscle mass and improve your capacity for exercise by reducing acidity in your muscles during high-intensity performance.
- **During-workout shake:** BCAAs (branched-chain amino acids) with a little creatine and sugar. BCAAs are found naturally in foods such as chicken, beef, tuna, salmon, whey and soy protein. For athletes, they prevent muscle soreness, fatigue and can help grow muscles. Creatine supplements are one of the most popular and effective supplements for improving strength, recovery and

muscle mass. It's also the most tested and safest supplement. Creatine is a substance that is found naturally in your muscles. Over 90 per cent of your body's creatine is stored within your muscles in the form of phosphocreatine, with the remaining 5 per cent or so found in your brain, liver and kidneys. When you take a creatine supplement, you increase your stores of phosphocreatine, which helps your body produce energy. Creatine should be consumed with some sugar, as sugar raises your insulin levels, which makes the creatine more effective at helping your muscles. For every 5 grams of creatine, you should take 70 grams of sugar. Sports juices can often provide this sugar.

- **Post-workout shake:** Dextrose in a supplement form, and a type of fruit for fructose. Dextrose is a sugar that digests very quickly, which means it will help fill your tank rapidly when you're running low on energy after a big exercise session.

- **Lunch:** Spicy curry or salmon cakes with spicy jalapenos, coriander (cilantro in the US) and Greek yoghurt. Salmon is full of lean, muscle-building protein and fatty omega-3 acids, which can reduce swelling in your muscles caused by lots of exercise. Coriander can actually reduce spasms and cramp.

- **Second lunch:** Skewered chicken with tzatziki sauce.
- **Dinner:** Red meat curry with turmeric. Red meat is rich in high-quality protein and in iron and zinc, minerals which can help athletic performance. Turmeric is a proven anti-inflammatory that has lots of health benefits, including preventing heart disease, some cancers and Alzheimer's. Some believe it can also help improve a number of the symptoms of depression.
- **Second dinner:** 'Power balls' made of almond butter, oatmeal, coconut, honey, pecans and dark chocolate chips rolled into balls. These are guilt-free hits of energy – without eating sweets!
- **Supper:** Honey Sriracha salmon on a bed of quinoa and Greek rice. Quinoa is high in fibre, protein and nutrients, and can help you lose weight as it can speed up your metabolism.

George sticks to lean meats to avoid extra saturated fat and cholesterol. He also cuts out processed sugar (the more sugar you eat, the more sugar you crave), substituting it with a teaspoon of cinnamon in a glass of hot water. To this he might add psyllium shells (a form of plant husks) to make it a high-fibre drink. Fat loss is a by-product of George's diet. However, his main objectives are better health, better performance and more strength and power.

Working with George has been like being promoted to the Premier League when it comes to food and nutrition. The ingredients are more sophisticated and are harder to find at the supermarket. But it's been worth the extra work in my opinion. George's food and approach to nutrition has reminded me that we are ultimately what we **think, do and eat**. The human gut has more neurons in it than there are in a cat's brain, which means your stomach is brainier than the next-door neighbour's moggy! That's reassuring. The health of your gut is directly connected with your brain, and the food you eat can affect your energy levels and how you feel about life. Below are some of the foods that will give you a boost of energy as well as making you feel good. They all find their way into my diet these days.

Mood and Energy Foods

- Bananas – a great source of potassium, which is an electrolyte that keeps the electricity, that ensures your heart carries on beating, flowing through your body. Bananas are also high in carbs and vitamin B6, which can improve brain function.

- Porridge – rich in vitamin B, fibre, iron and manganese, which can help your body with a slow release of energy.
- Fatty fish like salmon and tuna – these provide omega-3 and fight fatigue.
- Coffee – limited to a maximum of four cups per day, caffeine helps you keep alert.
- Brown rice – less processed than white rice, this contains fibre and minerals.
- Eggs – rich in amino acids, protein and vitamin B, and great fuel for the day ahead if you have them at breakfast.
- Apples – good for a slow energy release.
- Water – drinking regularly throughout the day avoids dehydration, which makes you feel sluggish.
- Sweet potatoes – a superfood bursting with vitamin A, which helps your eyesight, your immune system and your heart, lungs and other major organs.
- Yoghurt – protein-rich, and helps with a slow release of energy.
- Goji berries – high in fibre, low in sugar and low in calories, these sweet berries are called a superfood by some. According to some studies they can help improve your energy for exercise, improve your quality of sleep and keep you calmer.

- Avocados – another fibre-rich superfood, avocado is full of healthy fats and important nutrients. Avocados actually give you more potassium than bananas.
- Oranges – packed with vitamin C, oranges can boost your immune system and help your body's natural defences as an antioxidant.
- Green tea – another powerful antioxidant and stress fighter, green tea is a great alternative to coffee or normal tea.
- Nuts – high in fibre and carbs, and also good for slow energy release.

What Looks Good to You?

Remember, whatever looks good to you, doesn't necessarily look good to someone else. We're all different. So try not to worry what others think of you. And equally, avoid judging or labelling other people. You don't have to have a ripped body to be a good person or a fit one. After the weigh-in before my second fight with Wilder, some critics said I was too heavy, looked out of shape, and that Wilder was going to beat me easily. The truth was that only I knew how good I felt. And only I knew that I was at my perfect weight for that fight. The problem with today's world, particularly with social media because it's so visual, is that everything is about how we look. People try very hard to hold on to their younger looks and resist getting older. I say: go with it, forget your years and do your best to exercise, eat well and be happy! You might just become heavyweight champ, or reach any goal you want to.

CREATE YOUR OWN 'TRAINING CAMP': PREPARE YOURSELF FOR BRILLIANCE

FURIOUS WORKOUT IX

Wakey-wakey, rise and shine. Let's go for it and put our stamp on the day!

2 Minute Warm-up

- Jog on the spot for 20 sec
- Toe touches x 10
- Cross your legs, slowly touch toes for 10 sec x 2
- Bounce on the spot for 20 sec
- Swivel your hips for 20 sec, then the opposite way for 20 sec
- Kick legs out and shake for 10 sec

30 Minute Session

(3 x 10 min sessions)

- Jogging on the spot: left straight punch, right straight punch for 30 sec
- Jump squats x 15
- Press-ups x 12
- Sit-ups x 12
- Bicycle sit-ups x 12
- Half sit-ups/stomach crunches x 15
- Squats x 12
- Leg lunges x 12
- Burpees x 12
- Star jumps x 12

1 min break after each set. Then repeat. You'll notice there are more reps in each exercise here than in the last workout. If you're feeling exhausted, take a further break for 30 sec between exercises, then get back on it again. This is a tough one, but stick with it.

Warm-down

- Sit on floor, legs straight out, touch toes
- On floor, one leg straight, one leg in, touch toes for 10 sec then switch leg

- On floor, back straight, feet back and pressed together, push thighs down for 10 sec
- Standing up, pull one knee up, holding foot with hand, feel burn in thigh, switch leg
- Rotate hips for 30 sec then switch in other direction

Boxers have been going to training camps to prepare for fights for many years. As a fighter, when you head to a training camp, whether it's in the Rocky Mountains, Colorado, or in Runcorn, Cheshire, you know it's going to be tough, repetitious and at times even soul-destroying. But the old adage is so true: you get out what you put in. It is up to you. At my training camps my team and I look at who I am fighting, dissect their style and favourite tricks, and we plan accordingly. It is not only the place where I get physically fit, but it's also a kind of mental laboratory where I devise and then practise my strategy to beat my opponent, so come fight night it's simply a matter of execution.

In the five weeks before my training camp for the second Wilder fight, in Las Vegas, I was with my conditioner Kristian Blacklock, focusing on solidifying my body and building strength with high-resistance, low-volume training. Kristian then flew out with me and a close team (we'll get to them in a moment) for the eight-week camp itself. For those two months my week would typically look like this: two sessions of boxing every Monday, Tuesday, Thursday and Friday, with technical skills in the morning and sparring in the afternoon. To this, Kristian added core work and stretching. On Wednesday and Saturday, we did recovery running and more intense, explosive strength and conditioning.

Right up until the fight I was living cleanly. For example, in the past I used to eat a McDonald's after the weigh-in (to put on weight in the last twenty-four hours before a fight), but this time around I was more educated with my food, thanks to George Lockhart's input. Fast food is poor quality and processed, and to keep your motor going with that rubbish is akin to putting cooking oil in a Lamborghini. You deserve better; your stomach is less tolerant when you eat fatty food, and your energy levels suffer. But it wasn't just my diet for Wilder II that put me in the best position to win. For that fight I was in the best physical condition I have ever been in, and the training camp itself was perfect in so many ways. I've tried to nail down in this round what these keys to success were and have come up with a few transferable lessons which I hope you can integrate into your own life when you're preparing to face a big challenge.

Preparation

This first element is the whole point of a training camp: preparation. The more you can prepare for your challenge the more successful you are likely to be. Here are some fundamental questions you should ask yourself, which build on some of the other lessons we've learned so far in the book:

- What does success look like?
- Who or what is likely to block your path to success?
- How are you going to address/get rid of these roadblocks?
- Who do you need around you to help you succeed?

As we said earlier in the book, to be successful in any challenge in life you need to identify your goal, come up with a strategy to make it happen, establish the right routines to help you achieve that goal, and then adopt the right mindset.

The reason the Wilder II training camp was such a success was the clarity of our goal – we wanted to knock Wilder out and quickly. The strategy to achieve this was to coerce Wilder, put him on the back foot, dominate him with the extra weight I'd put on and wear him out with educated pressure, but the key component was increased punching power. In order to knock him out I was building the might and potency of my shots, and to make my punches more concussive I was hitting a heavy bag off its hook every day. The mastermind of my strategy for Wilder II was, of course, SugarHill Steward. Here's what SugarHill had to say about preparing me for the fight, and some tips for you too.

Coaching Advice from SugarHill Steward

'What work did I need to do to prepare Tyson for Wilder II? Everything was really already there. Tyson possesses every skill a good boxer should have. So talking to him is one of the main things I do with him, making sure he understands what talents he already has so that he realises his abilities. For a while nobody believed in him, but now they do.

'Understanding each other and communication is everything for a coach and their fighter. We don't talk boxing all the time, we talk like two pals. We talk about family, the past, present and future. We have to trust each other completely; he has to believe in what I can do and I have to believe in what he can do.

'Before we started working together I watched all of his previous fights. I knew that it wasn't enough to box to win; the only way he could guarantee to beat Wilder the second time would be to knock him out. I taught him that he needed to take control and leave the judges out of it; some of them would be for him, some of them against him. This is a lesson for life in general: don't leave fate to other people. Take control of it. I told Tyson he had the natural skills to tell himself: "The judges can throw their scorecards into the trash, I'm taking control and I'm going to knock him out." Ever since we talked about this he's now taking himself to a completely new level.

'A lot of what I do is psychological. Boxing is a mental game; a fighter who's not in shape but who has a fighter's instinct is stronger than a fighter who is in shape but mentally can't handle themselves. Being a Kronk-style fighter is about dominating the ring. It's not fancy, it's real simple and it's about going for the knockout. As Kronk boxers and coaches, we visualise it, then we go out and do it. You have to visualise success or it won't happen as you won't know where to go.'

Thanks, coach! As you can tell, it wasn't just SugarHill's strategy that I valued, it was his determination to achieve our shared goal. Of our training camp for Wilder II he said: 'All of the hard work and Tyson's dedication to the sport and his goal paid off. He wanted it. I wanted it too, just as much as he wanted it for himself.'

When I think back to most of my other training camps, compared with the one I put together for Wilder II, they were disorganised and a little shambolic. The one I experienced for the first Wilder fight seemed hexed from the beginning. Ten weeks before the fight we went to Big Bear training camp in California, which sits up in mountainous woods at an altitude of 7,000 feet. I'd never trained so high up in a place where the oxygen was so thin, and four weeks in, the place wasn't working for me. I felt terrible, couldn't breathe and I was tired all the time, be it on the bags, the pads or sparring. I just couldn't muster the energy I needed.

Nothing at all was going right, but I knew that on the night, if I could only get my mindset OK, I would prevail. Boxing is 99 per cent in the mind. My brother Shane suggested we go back down the mountain to LA and train there for the remaining four weeks. I was sceptical because I don't like changing camps. We rented a house and Freddie Roach, Manny Pacquiao's long-time coach, kindly welcomed us to his famous Wild Card gym in Hollywood. It took a week to get used to the new place and the sparring wasn't going well. I'd lost 10 stone in weight in a very short period. It was too much, too quickly, and in desperate protest, my body was flailing.

But I told myself: 'Sometimes, Mush, you just have to just roll with it.'

Preparing Your Mindset for Battle

As we've explored earlier in this book, I think that greatness is a mindset; everything is created in our minds. What you strive for and achieve in life comes from your having the right attitude to start with, the grit and determination to stay the course, and a finisher's guts to get all the way to your goal despite the difficulties encountered.

As you get nearer to achieving your goal, your mindset is more important than ever. It's no accident that all top sportsmen and women have similar mindsets, but the true champions are the ones who refuse to consider second place, who will give everything to win until the very last moments. When I was a kid, whether it was a football match, a running race, or even a competition to be the biggest idiot, I had to come first. I couldn't stomach anything less.

Floyd 'Money' Mayweather, one of the most successful boxers on the planet in terms of his unblemished fight record and the money he has earned from the game, is renowned for his unshakeable self-confidence. 'When I

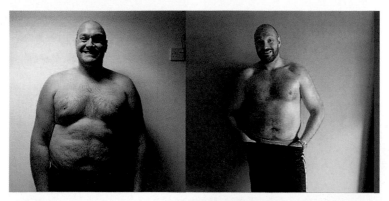

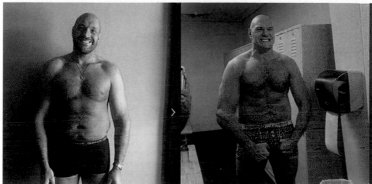

Top and middle: In the depths of my depression I weighed 28 stone. Thanks to exercise, eating more healthy food and the support of my friends and family I'm now in fighting fit shape at around 19 ½ stone.

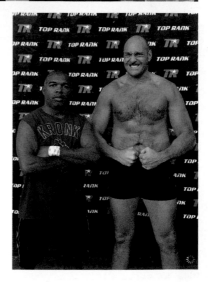

Right: With SugarHill before Wilder II.

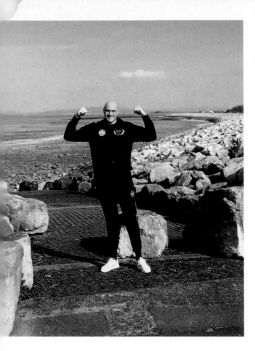

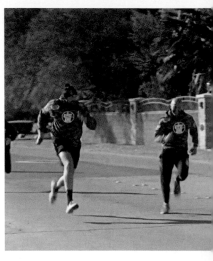

I love exercising outdoors. I enjoy running by the sea as the open horizon feels good for my spirit. Top left: Me at Morecambe Bay.

Sometimes I jog to local ruins, making my way through green fields, alongside stone walls and under huge skies. Below left: With my dad.

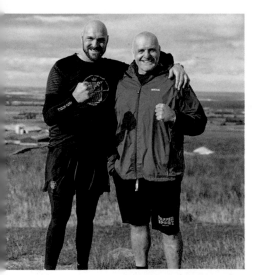

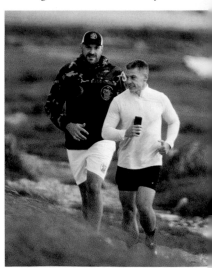

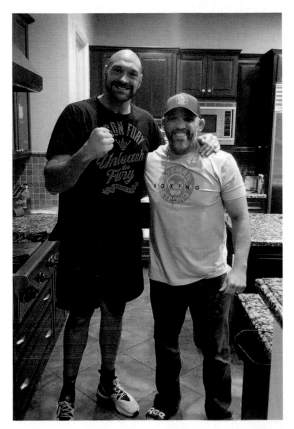

Before Wilder II, I contacted George Lockhart, the ex-US Marine turned MMA fighter, and now top nutritionist and chef to some of the world's best fighters. His formula is to eat moderate quantities of organic, healthy food consumed throughout the day in order to lose weight. I don't like vegetables much so George manages to hide them well in the meals he makes me.

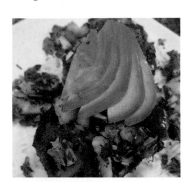 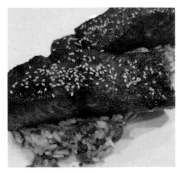

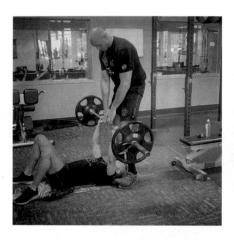

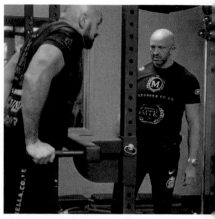

Two 'Old Baldy Heads'. In the gym with my strength and conditioning coach, Kristian Blacklock.
We do a range of upper body and lower body exercises, as well as high-intensity cardio.
Above: Kristian showing me floor bench presses, and me doing a tricep workout.
Below: Me doing a glutes exercise, and clap press-ups.

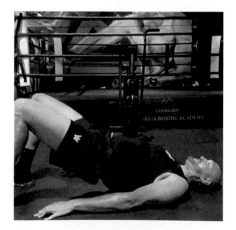

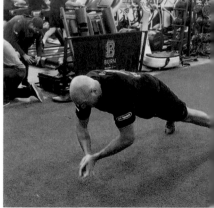

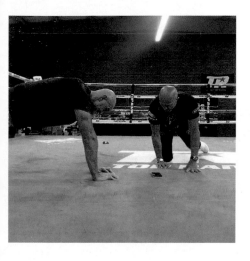
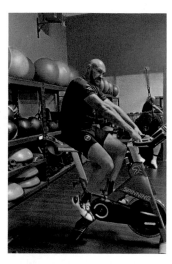

Above: Me doing a high plank, and warming down on the exercise bike.
Below: Building my upper body and explosive strength.

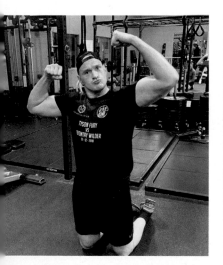
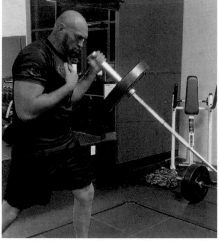

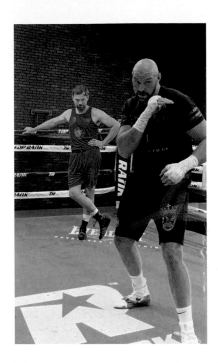
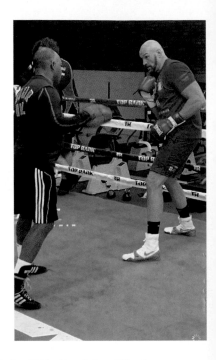

The 'sweet science'. Honing my aggressive boxing style before Wilder II, with SugarHill and boxer Andy Lee.

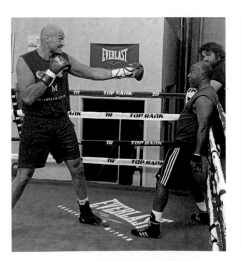
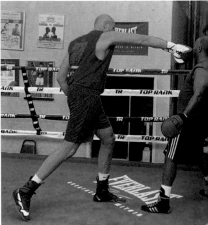

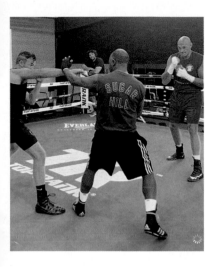

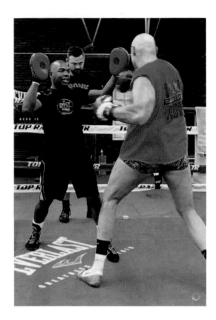

Above and below right: Everything went perfectly to plan in my Wilder II training camp. It all just clicked. Below left: A photo of me and the boys training in 2020 in the UK.

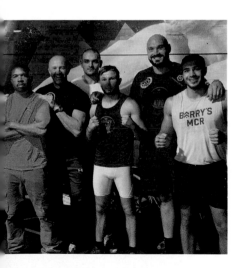

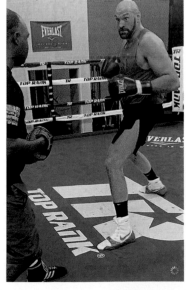

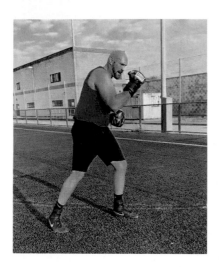

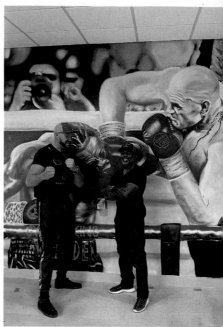

Above left: Training at the Tyson Fury Foundation gym in Morecambe. I hope it can inspire young people to get into sport.
Above right: During a training camp with SugarHill in 2020. Do you like the mural?
Below: An impromptu workout in Morecambe Bay in 2020. The future looks bright.

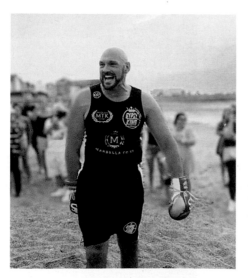

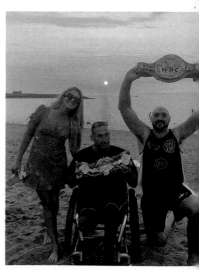

was a kid,' he says, 'I always thought I was a superstar.' He added: 'Before I turned professional, I thought I was the best and I kept believing it. And I knew eventually my hard work and dedication would pay off.' It's no surprise that he's famous for having brilliant training camps, and for getting his game face on early as he prepares in the lead-up to a fight. He has a high-performance winner's mindset.

Sugar Ray Leonard, one of the greatest ever craftsmen in boxing, says: 'The mental state of a boxer, and any other athlete or performer for that matter, is so significant and important in determining the outcome of a match. Nobody is born a champion just as no one is born a brain surgeon.'

As we've examined, it takes time to build the right mindset. Sugar Ray is a good example of this. When he missed out on going to the 1972 Olympics because he lost in the quarter-final of the trials, he was in floods of tears. But his assistant coach told him pointedly that he'd be more prepared and experienced come the next Olympics, and the young boxer – he was only sixteen at the time – took it all in.

From that moment on, Ray was purely focused on making the next Olympics and doing everything he could to bridge the gap. He would run five miles home behind the school bus, and then went straight to the gym. For the next four years he devoted himself to being a servant to his goal. And guess what? He made the next Olympic Games, in Montreal in 1976, and won gold.

Throughout the rest of Ray's career, things didn't always work out for him. He freely admits this was down to his mindset, which at times was more like a mind *upset*. 'When I lost my first professional fight, to Roberto Durán,' he said, 'I was devastated. Prior to Mike Tyson, Durán was the most intimidating fighter ever. He cursed me, he cursed my wife, he pushed me . . .' Durán had got into Ray's head, upset him on an emotional level and messed up his mindset. Instead of being the calm thinker he usually was in the ring, Ray got pulled into a machismo trap; fuelled by his personal rage against Durán, he tried to match the legendary Panamanian at streetfighting.

But Ray learned his lesson and come the rematch it was a very different story. He made a mockery of Durán's 'hands of stone' from the word go. This time he was thinking clearly as he danced, ducked and weaved and threw heavenly combos that left the Panamanian champion stupefied. Durán barely landed a punch before his own mindset crumbled in a fit of temper, refusing to fight on in the eighth round with the now infamous sentence, 'No más' (no more).

Speaking of mental preparation, Ray says: 'I block everything out so I get tunnel vision. I create the fight in my head. I see it, feel it, taste it. I talk to myself. You have to have belief in yourself.'

He has a neat little acronym which I think we can all live by:

P = Prepare
O = Overcome
W = Win
E = Every
R = Round

Ritual

Developing little rituals as you prepare for the final stages of your goal can also do wonders for your mindset. Like I said earlier, I like history, especially ancient history. Before a fight my team and I will come together in a circle to hug and say a prayer for both fighters. Sometimes we finish with the 'WE ARE SPARTA!' chant that I mentioned in the last round. I'll be honest, we got it from the film *300*. The film's a bit daft but good entertainment. What's important though is that this mantra has become an important ritual for us. Studies have shown that performing a familiar ritual before you enter into a stressful challenge or situation can lower your feelings of anxiety and even improve your performance, because you're more relaxed. When I shout like Gerard Butler does in *300* it puts a smile on my face and gets the adrenaline going. It's something we shout all the time in my training camps, so when fight night comes around, it's comforting and reassuring. It also reminds me once again of the real Spartans, ancient Greece's greatest fighting tribe. Like me they only knew fighting, as that was what their culture was based around and what they had dedicated themselves to. They were so practised in their preparation for warfare that cometh the hour, their mindset allowed them to fight their enemies with a quiet and lethal determination.

Try and think about what rituals you have in your own life, or any new rituals you can introduce. Remember, it's not all hocus-pocus or irrational thinking. Rituals can be a great tool for keeping your mindset positive, and they can become a safety blanket when you're in a tough situation or under pressure. It can help if your ritual is rooted in something that you can personally relate to, or that inspires you. When I think about the Spartans, I'm reminded of a funny story about them. Apparently the Persian King Xerxes once sent some spies to suss out the Spartans before a big battle, only for the spies to find them happily polishing their shields, oiling themselves up, stretching and doing gymnastics, as if they were relaxing.

The Spartan mindset was, *We're ready for you, bring it on.* Their elitism and sense of confidence over any challengers was not so different to the mindset of a world-beating athlete who believes absolutely in their ability, and whose thoughts are only fixed upon winning.

Sacrifice is Everything

In our training camps, a word we use a lot is 'sacrifice'. In high-level boxing it's small percentages that can make the difference between winning and losing. At the Vegas training camp in the lead-up to the second Wilder fight, I trained very hard and sacrificed more mentally and physically than I have ever done in my life. I was watching incredibly carefully what I ate and drank, going to bed early, waking up on time, pushing myself to the limit during my runs, my gym exercises and all of my boxing training, and I didn't skimp on the recovery either, with lots of massages and refuelling. I missed my family; by the time the fight came along I hadn't seen my wife and kids for ten weeks. But I knew the sacrifice would be worth it, and doing so much hard work and coming out the other side gave me huge confidence. Kristian remembers thinking he'd never seen an athlete at 100 per cent until that camp and I honestly think, even by my high standards, that I couldn't have done any more. I knew this was going to potentially be my career-defining fight, a fight which could cement who was the best heavyweight of this generation. I took away from myself things that I held dear, knowing that the rewards would be even greater.

I also knew that Wilder had been at home with his kids preparing for the fight and that he'd been drinking his soda and eating home-cooked food prepared by his aunt. Just the fact that he was in his comfort zone while I was out of mine stiffened my resolve. With Wilder II, I was in the best fettle I'd ever been in and for the first time in my boxing career I'd got everything right. If you get through any camp injury-free, it's a good indication it went well. Sometimes you get niggling injuries, sometimes serious ones. With all the media anticipation for Wilder II, and just as a cheeky way to see if there'd be any leaks from the circus following my camp (not from my team), I actually pretended to limp a little bit after one particular sparring session. Sure enough, suddenly there were rumours that I'd developed lots of injuries. I didn't mind if these rumours got out because I was feeling so good from all the sacrifices I'd made – and it was more mind games for Wilder to think about!

So dig deep to reach your goal; the sacrifices are worth it. You can't achieve anything without hardship.

Work With People You Trust and Respect

As I've said earlier in the book, whether you are an entrepreneur starting a business or a boxer preparing for a world-title fight, you are only as good as the sum of your parts – the people who make up your team. This is all the more important in a training camp, or in the final stages of preparation for your goal. To make everything work you need people who trust one another and share the same passion as you do for your goal. That can take time to achieve. I'm very careful about who I have around me at my training camp, and the golden rule is: only positive people. There are no lackeys and there's no big entourage in the Gypsy King camp, only a hand-picked, hard-working team who know what works for me and what doesn't. Most of us have been together for years now, so we all know what our roles are and work like a well-oiled machine. They understand me and my down moods and I can be honest with them. The Las Vegas Wilder II team included:

- **SugarHill Steward** my main coach
- **Andy Lee** second coach
- **George Lockhart** nutritionist

- **Kristian Blacklock** strength and conditioning coach
- **Isaac Lowe** my training partner
- **Timothy Alcock** organiser
- **Shane** and **Hughie** my brothers

Easy/Rapid Communication

What was great about my team was not only that they all knew their roles, they also knew not to step on anyone else's toes. SugarHill and Kristian, for example, worked seamlessly together and communicated constantly so they could be on the same page. Both are experts in their own fields and apply their knowledge of the ring and physiology to me and my body with the precision of scientists. SugarHill would tell Kristian exactly what he had been working on so he knew which of my muscles would already have been worked. Just as George, my nutritionist, knew when I needed a nourishing pick-me-up between exercises and was in constant dialogue with Kristian. I also had my regular training partner and good friend Isaac Lowe, who is the WBC International featherweight champion, on hand. We have a great dynamic and that added good familiarity. Having my second cousin Andy Lee as second coach was another a big positive. Andy was an excellent boxer in his own right, a former world middleweight champion who only hung up his gloves in 2017. Since then he's coached some very promising up-and-coming Irish boxers. Again, I trust him and we're on the same wavelength when we talk to each other so nothing gets lost in communication.

If you have a team of diverse talents, make sure they are all pulling in the same direction, with one primary goal made up of smaller goals. Our overarching goal was to win the WBC heavyweight title via achieving smaller goals leading up to the event: good diet, great conditioning, getting enough rest, making sure my mindset was in the right place, working on my concussive punches and aggression. Everybody played their part.

Look After Your Team and They'll Look After You

The sparring was particularly good at the Wilder II camp. We had some really sharp, hungry boxers. Some days at camp I would spar with four different partners. Each one would come in fresh to do a round, with me going full-tilt. Four first rounds are a killer for anyone! Training with a seasoned pro like me is a great opportunity for young fighters on the way up. They're fresh and hungry and give me the best workout because they're not just turning up for a payday, they want to work and learn. They're also looking to knock you out. I only ever ask for fighters who will try and do that.

In return I properly look after them. I pay them well, put them in the best accommodation possible, give them money for food and entertainment. I look after them so well because they are vital keys in unlocking my potential in the camp. At the end of the day they're there to help me so I've got to take care of them.

Getting Enough Sleep and Rest

Another key element of a boxing training camp is ensuring you get the right rest and preparation, and that means going to bed early. This applies to all of us in life. If we don't sleep well, we won't perform at our best, whatever our goals. As we discussed earlier in the book, sleep is essential for the brain to have time to relax and process what its learnt and also to work through things that may be worrying your mind. It's also the time when your body best repairs itself and creates greater physical resilience for the next day.

For me in camp, there's no running around between training, no leaving the house. After training and eating, it's about resting properly, putting my feet up, playing computer games maybe, fully relaxing and then sleeping. It's basically train, eat, rest and sleep, repeat.

But how to sleep before a big fight, or a big moment in your life? I'm not worried about getting hurt the next day. It's the winning or losing factor, the need to perform because there's a lot on the line, that used to keep me up, particularly in my early career, when I was still an amateur. To counter those thoughts, these days I try to get plenty of rest the day before and relax on the day of the fight. While Paris is nervous before a fight in case I get hurt, I mostly have a sense of inner calm, created from the confidence generated in my camp. If everybody had an ability like this not to get nervous in fights, they'd all be world champions. I think my relaxation before fights (and then later in the ring) is unusual. I never really get flustered before a fight because I love doing what I do. It's my moment: all the lights will soon be on me. I've done all the hard work, I've trained for this moment, I've done it all my life, and I will get well paid for it. As I said earlier in the book, I used to get nervous as an amateur but not now as a professional. Putting everything into perspective like this definitely helps.

In the same way, if you've got a big day of any kind coming up, perhaps a job interview, or an important presentation, make sure you go to bed knowing that you have done all the preparation you need to, that you've covered every base. This will help you sleep well the night before. Try to think about everything that has led you to that moment, and take confidence from your journey. If you do have anxieties that are preventing you sleeping (in the day or weeks before you achieve your goal), talk about your problems with yourself and others and try to plan for that contingency. To prevent you from just lying there worrying, write down the problem or problems, then add what measures you might take so your mind can relax. Make sure you're eating and drinking well, too. An unhealthy diet can sometimes make sleep harder. By contrast, some foods actually contain sleep-promoting substances. These include bananas, honey, seeds, nuts, eggs and dairy. So remember: plan, work hard, relax, eat well, and then go to bed, you dosser!

Keeping Distractions at Bay

As we've established, when you're in the final stages of your goal, you need the right environment in which to be your best. This also means cutting out superfluous noise and distractions. In boxing, protecting the athlete from things that don't concern him or her, like the media, is important. The promoter's job is to sell the fight as much as possible, and they'd have you doing interviews all day and every day in fight week if they could. So it's up to your team to keep the promoter at bay so you can focus on your goal. Like a Grand National-winning racehorse, the prize fighter must be worked out, well looked after, pampered, massaged, washed down, fed and watered, and put to bed with nice clean bedding. Having a contrast between work and play is also essential.

I once heard that the boxer Marvin Hagler created a self-styled prison at the Provincetown Inn in Cape Cod. The only other guests allowed were his sparring partners. 'There's nothing but concentration,' he said. He used loneliness as a way to ignite his inner rage. 'You're supposed to seclude yourself. All the great champions did the same. Rocky Marciano, Ali up on his mountain at Deer Lake. They put themselves in jail. I put myself in jail.'

I don't go quite that far. I like to go to jail, but with a few close family and team members! Marvellous Marvin was a loner without any company. For me it's important that I have my brothers and my team. I hate being alone. I'm an outgoing person and need the stimulus of others around me. So after training we'll play pool, chill out in the hot tub or swimming pool, play some table tennis. With all the hard work there has to be some downtime. I've got to have banter with the boys, and have fun conversations. One minute we might be chatting about whether Pringles are actually a crisp or a cracker (a debate I had with my brothers in the Wilder II camp when I was on the massage table) and the next minute we could be talking about ancient dynasties: the Egyptians, the ancient Greeks, the Romans, the Babylonians . . . each had their moment in the sun then eventually vanished, as is the case with boxers I suppose. With my team we like to talk about great fighters, too, from Muhammad Ali to Mike Tyson; we're all schooled in the history of boxing. No two conversations are the same.

Although I have the camaraderie of those around me in camp, I find it very hard, like any father and husband would do, to be apart from my family and kids. But I know that it will only be temporary, and it will be worth the sacrifice. I'm a family man and I love nothing more in the world than my wife and kids, but in order to do my job and to put money in the bank and food on the table I have to go away and put my fighting head on. Whatever your goal is, make sure you give it the best chance.

That Little Bit Extra is What Makes a Winner

I've said it before, but in all walks of life, it's those who dig their heels in and go the extra mile who prevail. Not the most talented, but those with grit and determination. For what is talent without consistency and application? High-level boxing is not for tourists who briefly dip in and give it a go. It's for those prepared for a long, hard road ahead. It's the same for any goal in life. You have to fully commit. Nobody can make you get up in the morning while it's still dark and force you to go running, or to do the extra work to start your business. Nor can anyone make you dig deep and win fights, nor make you find the mental strength to stay at the negotiating table to land a difficult deal. It's all about your inner drive.

You Get Back What You Put In

At the start of this round I said that the key to any training camp is that you get out what you put into it. This holds true for any goal or challenge you prepare for in life. It's short-term pain for long-term gain. Muhammad Ali once said: 'I hated every minute of training, but I said [to myself], "Don't quit. Suffer now and live the rest of your life as a champion."' Remember those words when you're toughing it out in training, or working on a goal that seems impossible. The difference between winning or losing really is granular. It's all about the smallest of margins.

DISTRACTIONS: HOW TO BLOCK OUT THE HATERS

FURIOUS WORKOUT X

Get up! Anything is possible today. You can do it!

2 Minute Warm-up

- Jog on the spot for 20 sec
- Toe touches x 10
- Cross your legs, slowly touch toes for 10 sec x 2
- Bounce on the spot for 20 sec
- Swivel your hips for 20 sec, then the opposite way for 20 sec
- Kick legs out and shake for 10 sec

30 Minute Session

(3 x 10 min workouts)

- Left/right straight punches running on the spot x 60
- Static jump lunges x 15
- Jump squats x 15
- Clap press-ups x 5
- Sit-ups x 15
- Bicycle sit-ups x 15
- Plank for 30 sec
- Squats x 15
- Leg lunges x 15
- Star jumps x 15

1 min break after each set. Then repeat. If you're feeling knackered, you can take a further break for 30 sec between exercises.

Warm-down

- Sit on floor, legs straight out, touch toes
- On floor, one leg straight, one leg in, touch toes for 10 sec, then switch leg
- On floor, back straight, feet back and pressed together, push thighs down for 10 sec
- Standing up, pull one knee up, holding foot with hand, feel burn in thigh, switch leg
- Rotate hips for 30 sec then switch in other direction

In Rounds Five and Six, I told you about some of the times during my life when I went so far as to move to new places to get rid of old habits, and other points when I stopped hanging around with certain people – or 'negative dossers' as I call them – who were a bad influence on me and my journey to recovery. Similarly, as we examined in the last round with training camps, it's crucial that during the final stages of preparing for a goal there aren't too many distractions competing for your attention.

Blocking out naysayers, standing up to bullies and controlling the controllables are things I want to look at in more detail now. If you can find the strength to ignore people who are only trying to tear you down, it's such a liberating feeling. Instead of trying to please others, you will feel empowered if you can live fully for yourself for the first time. Once you start to live this way, alongside embracing failure and learning from your own mistakes, you'll soon be able to triumph over almost any situation. And you'll definitely need these skills when reaching for your greatest goals.

Blocking Out the Haters

When someone feels inferior to, jealous of, or hateful towards you, but is unable to be straight up with their misgivings, it often gets communicated in a subtle, passive-aggressive style. This is done in a way that doesn't directly show the toxic nature of the behaviour, but it can still make you question yourself, your ability and even your hopes. Insinuations and leading questions are often the tools people use to chip away at your confidence. For instance, someone might say: 'You know it's going to be very difficult to be successful doing what you're doing. Do you think maybe you could do something which was more likely to work?'

Doubters can prevent the green shoots of your ambition from flourishing. How many dreams have been rubbished because someone else felt threatened by another's passion and conviction? Even some people you consider to be friends may limit your vision or tell you that you are not being realistic because they are unable to imagine reaching such heights themselves, or are threatened by your possible success. And there are those who try to make you feel bad about your success. All I can say is that I don't take any of it personally; their doubts are probably rooted in their own problems, not mine. Don't allow their behaviour to seed self-doubt in yourself; don't descend to that level. When faced with haters, doubters and naysayers, I try to be compassionate and ask myself why they are behaving like that, and what's gone wrong for them that they can be so angry about nothing.

We all have different skills and talents. Maybe they are frustrated with their lot so their frustration in themselves finds an outlet by knocking what I have achieved. The most important thing is not to lose sight of your intention and self-worth. But at the same time, sometimes you need to put the blinkers on, like on a horse, to block out the negativity of others.

Think Like Arnie

Someone I admire is Arnold Schwarzenegger. On YouTube there's a video of a speech he gave on success, where he says: 'When you hear the naysayers, don't doubt yourself. Don't think about having a Plan B. Because having a Plan B will take away your energy for Plan A. Plan B is a safety net, and we know that people perform better when there is no Plan B. And why do they need a Plan B? Because they are afraid of failing.'

When he first tried to break into acting, Arnie was ridiculed for his accent and his muscular body. But Arnie had the last laugh over his critics when James Cameron cast him in *The Terminator*, which became a massive box-office hit. Cameron said to the press: 'If Arnold hadn't have had the body and talked like a machine, I think the movie wouldn't have worked.' So Arnie's weakness as perceived by others was actually his greatest asset. What do our doubters really know?

When I ballooned to 28 stone and was suffering ill mental health, I was written off (and probably with good reason) by journalists and athletes who said I'd never come back. But I did. And when it was announced I would face the world's most dangerous boxer, a lot of people thought the Wilder fight was too much too soon, while others said I was a feather-duster puncher who didn't have a chance. When people doubt me I always produce the goods; their doubt drives me on.

Don't give your doubters and their opinions any weight, instead follow your own path and have faith in yourself. It's good to put egg on people's faces; success is so much sweeter when you prove your doubters wrong. As Arnie says, when someone says *impossible*, you say *possible*; when they say *can't*, you say *can*. Remember Nelson Mandela's inspiring advice: 'It always seems impossible until it's done.'

Tips for Blocking Out Haters

- Try to ignore them
- Try to avoid them in the first place
- Don't validate their behaviour with a response

- Try and understand why they are acting the way they are
- If you can't ignore them and if they keep making you feel bad, confront them about how they are making you feel

If someone dishes out a negative comment to you, recycle it as a signal to recommit to your work and to refocus on the road ahead of you. And if you're going to confront somebody about the way they are acting, make sure you have a cool head and a warm heart; don't launch into the conversation with pent-up aggression. Life is too short. Be calm, say what you need to say and keep it neutral.

In Morecambe I live in my own self-created bubble of sunshine. As much as I can I've tried to design my life so that it's a positive one of friends, family and a firm routine of training. Anything that is going to make me feel crap I've removed and put as far away as possible. I'd rather keep myself to myself than be brought down by external negative vibes.

Social Networking is an Addiction

Fact. Social networking is a dangerous animal and can have a negative effect on your self-esteem, with perfect strangers trolling you for no reason. It's sad that a person we've never met can post a comment that makes us look stupid or shames us in front of thousands or even millions of others. Social network bullying is brutally ugly; someone chipped away at over a period of time can feel very alone in their persecution; it can drive us to depression or worse.

One trick on Instagram I've found is to turn off the comments so no one can reply. In that way I can post something positive, like my lockdown fitness videos, but then I don't have to read any negativity that might come through and ruin my day. Social media is good for letting the world know what you're up to, but if you start reading comments, you start to over-think. On my site I don't allow messages from people I don't know.

I worry about young people spending so much time on these platforms and the pain they're opening themselves up to. It's more subtle than we might realise. Some of the nerds in Silicon Valley who designed this stuff have admitted they knew how addictive it would become (they even keep it away from their own children). The whole thing works on a reward system, like the one invented by that scientist, Doctor Pavlov, who rang a bell each time he fed his dogs. The dogs got so used to the bell representing mealtimes that in the end they salivated just on hearing the bell, even when there was no food; just as we've got used to feeling so good about receiving a 'like' or a 'love' symbol each time we put a photo of ourselves on our page. These symbols represent being accepted by others and fitting in with them, and our brains release dopamine reward hits as a result. And while we seek out reward 'likes' from perfect strangers to make ourselves feel socially accepted, Silicon Valley are busily using algorithms to track what we like and who we follow, so they can pass on this information to companies who want to influence us.

What kind of world are we living in when people base their self-esteem on how many likes they get and how many followers they have? We shouldn't be defined by our looks, but rather the person we are inside. As my pal Shaun says, when kids are Photoshopping their faces to look perfect, something has gone very wrong. Mental-health problems built on inferiority complexes have gone through the roof since the introduction of Instagram, Snapchat, Twitter, YouTube, TikTok and Facebook.

If you're getting bullied online this could be a criminal offence. Know your rights: you can report this to the police. If someone abused you on the street they could potentially get arrested, and fortunately cybercrimes are now being taken more seriously. If social media is getting you down on a less serious level, try to get away from your phone, remove yourself from the situation, so this abuse can't touch you, can't hurt you. You wouldn't willingly let hyenas into your house would you? So shut the cyber gate and don't give social media a chance to sink its claws in.

Bullies

Belittling someone else to make yourself feel better about your own shortcomings is as old as time. There are many different kinds of bullying, including online trolling as we've just discussed. But the common denominator about bullies is that they are all insecure inside. When I was in Year 3 at primary school I was bullied by kids in Year 6 because I was tall and lanky; I guess maybe they were jealous and felt vertically challenged on some level. Bullies, I've found, fold when you take it to them or get help to confront them, because although they prey on the weak, they're not strong people themselves.

Peer pressure is very common these days, and that too is a form of bullying. Often people who are a little bit different in how they look or think are targeted by the herd. Just because everybody else is doing something, that doesn't make it OK.

If you're bullied at school or at work, speak to your teachers, your boss or your colleagues. There will be formal complaint procedures in place to help protect you as no one has the right to do this to you. If you can confront your bully and you feel safe to do so, tell them that they're causing you mental or emotional damage. If you don't feel like there's anyone you know you can turn to, there are bullying helplines you can call and charitable organisations that can support you and give you advice on what you can do. Remember: sometimes we have to fight for what's right. This doesn't mean getting your fists out. It means standing up, knowing it's not your fault, and that you're not on your own. Not everyone has guts naturally but at some stage in life we may all have to confront bullies. Even if you think you are the biggest coward in the world, know that we all have the potential to dig deep, stand up for ourselves and find our courage to face those who are in the wrong. You can do it.

Choose What is Worth Worrying About

I mentioned earlier in the book that my friend Shaun Gash has helped to teach me to only worry about things that I can control, and to put other doubts out of my mind. With the world in such a strange and scary state at the moment it can be hard to do this because it feels like we're teetering on the edge of a very unstable future. Whether it's the Covid-19 pandemic, the wildfires in California eating up forests the size of Leeds every day, or the growing gap between the rich and the homeless, no wonder we feel anxious about what will happen to our parents, our jobs, the struggling companies we work for, and our kids' educations. It's natural that mental-health problems are growing. But in the face of all of this, we must try to keep Shaun's advice in our minds about only choosing to worry about what we can control.

Control the Controllables

Try this exercise below to test what's really in your grasp.

1. Write down on a sheet of A4 everything that is worrying you about the past, the present and the future. It could be anything: paying the mortgage, the Covid-19 pandemic, the state of politics, a health problem or relationship issues. Whatever it is, mush, get it all down on paper

2. Rewrite the worry list with your most pressing worries at the top, going down to the lesser worries at the bottom of the list

3. On a third sheet of paper now list the items you have any control over

In all likelihood the final list of worries you can control is very small compared to the first list of all your worries. For example, you can attempt to bridge the gap in your relationship with your spouse but you can't ultimately control what goes on in their head. You can go and see the doctor about the lump you've found, but you have no final say over whether it's malignant or harmless. You can work hard at your job but you can't control if the business is going to go under because of a pandemic or other external global factors. Like I said earlier in the book, the one thing you can control is how you react to these worries and fears. People act negatively because of all sorts of fears: fear of failure, fear that others' success will make them look like failures, fear of change, fear of what if. If you can prioritise your worries you can control your fear, and you can live more positively.

Turn it Off!

Have you ever noticed what happens when you don't watch the news because you're on holiday, or are in the middle of nowhere so can't get a copy of a newspaper?

Nothing. Nothing happens and the world keeps turning. You don't need to be plugged in to the negativity. Actually, something does happen: you begin to feel better, less troubled by the background noise of worry. Because that's what it is, background noise that quietly builds into anxiety. With a constant barrage of newsfeeds on our phones, twenty-four-hour news on our TVs and pop-up breaking news on our social media, it's no wonder that we've learnt to live in a constant state of low-level stress. It's not good for you; not for your heart, your thoughts, your energy levels or your soul. Stress ages you. The solution is to stop the toxic stuff getting into your mind by reducing your screen-time on your phone, tablet or laptop and only occasionally watching the news.

We don't realise how precious and brief our time on this planet is until we're old. You don't want to look back on your life and realise you've wasted time worrying about things you couldn't change. Life is to be lived and enjoyed.

BUILDING YOUR OWN ALTER-EGO AND CHANNELLING YOUR HEROES

FURIOUS WORKOUT XI

You should be feeling the benefits of all these workouts by now! Hang in there. Let's get ready to rumble and go again!

1 Minute 50 Second Warm-up

- Jog on the spot for 20 sec
- Cross your legs, slowly touch toes for 10 sec x 2
- Bounce on the spot for 20 sec
- Swivel your hips for 20 sec, then the opposite way for 20 sec
- Punches on the spot for 10 sec

30 Minute Session

(3 sets)

- Jump squats x 20
- Plank for 30 sec
- Sit-ups x 20
- Bicycle sit-ups x 20
- Squats x 20
- Half sit-ups/stomach crunches x 20
- Leg lunges x 20
- Burpees x 20
- Star jumps x 20
- Tricep lifts x 20 (find a chair, a low wall or bench and put your legs out in front of you, with your feet planted on the floor. Slowly raise your body up and down using your triceps to lift you and lower you)

1 min break after each set. Then repeat. If your abs are hurting, it's probably working! But don't push through too much pain. You can take a further 30 sec break between exercises if it's too much.

Warm-down

- Sit on floor, legs straight out, touch toes
- On floor, one leg straight, one leg in, touch toes for 10 sec then switch leg

- On floor, back straight, feet back and pressed together, push thighs down for 10 sec
- Standing up, pull one knee up, holding foot with hand, feel burn in thigh, switch leg
- Rotate hips for 30 sec then switch in other direction

The Gypsy King is a persona, no different from Bruce Wayne and his alter ego, Batman. The Gypsy King is nothing like the real me, but I couldn't be the world champ without him. He's fearless, cocky, loud and showy, whereas I fall prey to the same doubts about myself as anyone else, probably more so because of my up and down psyche. The Gypsy King oozes charisma and sticks his tongue out like a Maori warrior. Whereas I enjoy making a nice cup of tea and playing with the dog. He can hold sold-out arenas in the palm of his hand, making them laugh or belting out American ballads. OK, I still belt out songs at home! But Paris could never live with the Gypsy King. And neither could I.

Sometimes you can get lost in your own hype, like actors who play hard-men roles for so long that they end up thinking they're dangerous. For a while earlier in my career, as I wrote about in *Behind The Mask*, I did get a bit lost with the crazy character I was playing in boxing. But these days I don't blur the line. Although I have nothing but respect for the Gypsy King when I'm in the boxing world, I know that I'm ultimately the boss. I only bring him out when he's required, in order for me to perform at my top level as a fighter and as a showman.

Now, you might not need an alter ego for every situation. Arriving at work in a crown and cape sitting on top of a throne might give the wrong impression! But creating a bullet-proof persona to make you feel confident in order to get you through high-pressure moments in your life is something that we can all benefit from. And that's what we're going to explore in this round.

I'm not the first and I won't be the last person to adopt a persona. We've all done it, probably when we were kids, play-acting and pretending we were someone else with special powers or superhuman skills. In boxing and wrestling it's obviously very common for fighters to have a stage name or nickname, partly to help build the drama, and so the crowd can root for different 'characters'. The difference now is that play-acting has the respectable rubber stamp of psychologists and performance coaches who are studying it across lots of different individuals and fields. A bloke called Todd Herman, who is an award-winning performance expert, even wrote a book called *The Alter Ego Effect*, in which he explores the idea that some of the greatest actors, athletes and world figures throughout history have used this strategy very successfully to effectively become someone else.

Apparently Winston Churchill wore different hats – from top hats to bowlers – to help bring out different personalities within himself that would help him overcome challenges, depending on the room he was walking into, or the situation at hand.

I think this all makes a lot of sense. If there is a trait in your personality or an item in your mental tool-box that's missing – say a behaviour, a characteristic, or an attitude – then by adopting an alter ego you can summon another self where all the missing parts of your identity are added in. An alter ego or persona is someone other than the day-to-day you; the person you would like to be in certain situations where you are otherwise lacking.

Alter egos are often 'bigger' versions of yourself. If you were to walk out onto a stage in front of tens of thousands of people, to capture everyone's attention you would need to be commanding and free from fear or stage fright. By becoming a supreme version of yourself, who moves and talks in a different way, you can overcome your own self-doubting personality, and take on a more confident character.

The Gypsy King has been with me since I was about ten years old, when I used to persuade my dad to take me to the gym where he trained as a boxer. He'd buy me a McDonald's and I'd sit in the corner chomping through it. Then I'd be up on my feet shadow boxing, throwing shapes. The awkward, shy and lanky kid who was picked on by older boys began to develop another self. The ring felt very much like home; I had a natural affinity with learning punch combinations. Boxing gloves just felt right on my hands. When I started fighting in organised bouts I felt like a straight-backed, stronger, more relaxed version of myself and I was utterly assured of my own talent. Being descended from two undefeated 'Gypsy Kings' – real titles given to the top fighter in the Travellers community – I was aware of my family's heritage and pedigree. I even knew the Irish songs. So that made me feel like fighting royalty in these boxing situations. The character began to grow from there, and I felt very confident and comfortable with him when I got into the ring.

Next time you watch me fight on TV, notice how easy and calm I am; how I seem to be 'in the moment', from before the fight in the dressing room, to the ring walk, and then once the fight begins. The Gypsy King has taken over. It's his show. And I feel bigger than any man, and capable of anything. Before Wilder II I was so relaxed in the dressing room that I was blowing kisses to Wilder when they cut to the TV screens showing both fighters.

While all this might sound a bit like I'm blowing smoke up my arse, I really do believe alter egos can help us achieve amazing things. When I am 'him' I fear nothing, and that's quite handy in my line of business. The Gypsy King gets turned on when I need him, and turned off as soon as his job is done. This alter ego has developed quite naturally for me. But apparently coaches across America are now intentionally identifying mental, physical and even social traits that their athletes are lacking, and then creating tailor-made alter egos to take their athletes to the next level in performance.

Another history lesson now. Apparently in Roman times there was a concept called modelling – and no, it didn't involve walking down a catwalk. The idea was that you could choose role models to base your behaviour on. They might be great military leaders or great thinkers, whatever floated your boat. Once you'd mapped out what it was about the person you wanted to mimic, then you set about trying to live up to their standards.

Alexander the Great was obsessed with following in the footsteps of Achilles, the greatest warrior of the ancient Greeks, who slayed Hector during the Trojan War. Alexander visited his hero's tomb in modern-day Turkey and paid homage there, as well as having Achilles' motto above the entrance to his tent, which translates to something close to 'Be the best and far above all others.' He certainly succeeded in that: by the age of thirty he had conquered a quarter of the world.

Two centuries on, Julius Caesar was obsessed with

Alexander and modelled himself on many of his actions. Just as Alexander was the first in to battle on his black horse, and was loved by his men for fighting with them rather than hiding in a tent far away from the battlefield, Caesar was respected by his troops for fighting alongside them. While on campaign, he'd sleep rough under the stars with his men, covered only by his shield.

As we grow up we all have heroes who we imitate, whether it's pop stars, astronauts, actors or comic-book characters. So the idea that we channel the behaviour of another is nothing new. It's another form of play-acting when you think about it, something we used to do naturally as kids before we learnt to be self-conscious and had to grow up. The trick is trying to keep this talent for imagination and play-acting alive as an adult, so you can use it to help bring out your inner hero in tough moments, or on the journey to achieving your goal. If you're on a quest to lose weight, having a super 'you' who doesn't cave in and eat all the cookies in the house is a good ally to have.

Many of us have a fear of failure, and when your identity, especially as a sportsperson, is so closely tied to your success in your chosen field, it makes losing a very big problem. However, when you hand over responsibilities to an alter ego, you can pass on that fear of failure; you can get rid of it. The alter ego also helps sportspeople avoid an identity crisis when they are forced to retire. We can with a little effort construct newer and better versions of ourselves. So if you're facing challenges and major obstacles in progressing towards your ultimate goal, start by thinking about the kinds of qualities you need to succeed. If you're shy, you might need to take on more extroverted traits. It's essentially a challenge to your mindset. Once you've identified the behaviour you want, you can create a persona who will inhabit this behaviour.

We can all learn to adopt new traits and step into the shoes of excellence to get into 'the zone' completely focused on the challenge or the task at hand. It's a place where we can break free of our previous self-limiting doubt and fear. Just as Alexander made a tribute to Achilles in order for him to receive his courage and blessing in the next battle, we lesser mortals have little rituals we practise before an important event to invoke our alter egos. Some wear a lucky, talismanic T-shirt under their office shirt, or lucky undies, while others have an item they clutch. Personally, I say a prayer before I go in the ring; everybody is different.

I hear Deontay Wilder meditates before a fight to summon and channel his alter ego, the spirit of a Nigerian ancestor warrior. He believes it's a completely different entity to himself: 'When I turn into the Bronze Bomber it separates me from other fighters. I get a scary feeling when I turn into him. I become stronger.'

Wilder and I are not the first fighting men to create a persona and we won't be the last. My dad named me after the most feared fighter of all time. In terms of explosive punching power doubled with killer instinct, 'Iron Mike' Tyson was unprecedented; he put even the likes of George Foreman and Sonny Liston in the shade. But though he was a naturally aggressive, physical fighter he wasn't the finished article and one day his trainer, Cus D'Amato, said that he wished Mike was bigger. It hit Mike deep. Mike admitted that he wasn't emotionally invested in being the villain Cus wanted him to be before then. But that comment about him being too small spurred him on. Mike immersed himself in the bad-guy characters in movies and focused on becoming like them. Mike revealed that, out of the ring, he was totally afraid of everything; of losing, of being humiliated. But he said that the closer to the ring he got, the more confident he became: 'Once I'm in the ring I'm a god, no one can beat me.'

Tyson channelled the American boxer Jack Dempsey too. 'Dempsey . . . wanted to maim you. He didn't want you dead. He wanted you to suffer. He wanted to shatter your eye socket, destroy your cheeks, your chinbone. That's what I learnt from Mr Dempsey and I believe I learnt it well.' The problem is Iron Mike began to trespass into Mike's own life. 'I thought being a feared person was a respected person,' he said.

David Bowie, the ultimate chameleon of the twentieth century, created Ziggy Stardust in order to break out of ten years of limited success as Davy Jones from Beckenham. He later became David Bowie and wrote some great albums but he still wasn't where he knew he deserved to be. It wasn't until Bowie cut his long locks off, dyed them bright orange, put on a dodgy-looking skin-tight space suit and became Ziggy Stardust (who hailed not from Kent but from the other side of the cosmos) that Bowie came to hold the world in his palm. He was an overnight success ten years in the making. But there was a problem: Bowie got a little too good at being Ziggy, or did Ziggy get too good at being him? He wasn't able to turn him off after a performance and Ziggy's drug intake went through the stratosphere. Bowie publicly killed him off at the end of a tour. It's important to create boundaries for your alter ego: by handing over the blame and responsibility to one you run the risk of it taking you over.

Of the fabulous 'Four Kings' of boxing – Marvin Hagler, Roberto Durán, Sugar Ray Leonard and Thomas 'Hitman' Hearns – three had alter egos. Leonard looked into a mirror before each fight and if he saw Sugar Ray looking back at him he knew he couldn't lose. However, if he saw average Ray Leonard, then the odds were against him. He even had a second alter ego. When he got in trouble he unleashed the 'Streetfighter'. When Leonard first fought Hearns, although Sugar Ray showed up in his refection, he still felt an uncontrollable fear creep into his mind, but then he saw Muhammad Ali in the audience and channelled him, becoming 'the Greatest' for the fight. As Ali he was unbeatable, and because Ray knew Ali wouldn't have been scared of Hearns, neither was he. After the fight he said: 'I couldn't have stopped even if I'd wanted to. The exhilaration as each shot met its target, the most wonderful feeling in the world. I fed off the roar of the fans and the sign of my opponent in trouble.'

Hearns would talk about the 'Hitman' in the third person, as if he was a separate person, while Hagler believed he had a monster inside him that made him scream like a madman while he was in training. Durán? I guess he was a beast in his default setting. He didn't need to channel his aggression!

There are lots of tales of musicians who became successful after developing alter ego personas. Calvin Cordozar Broadus Jr found a lot more fame as Snoop Dogg; Christopher Wallace became a legend as Biggie Smalls and the Notorious B.I.G. Alter egos allow us to step out of our comfort zones and become someone else that we want to be. They help us take risks and bridge the gap between where you are and where you ideally want to be.

How to Build Your Alter Ego

Why do you want to create an alter ego? What is your goal? Be clear about the skills you need to adapt to achieve your goal. Write them down. What is it you want your alter ego to be? More relaxed, more self-assured, or more authoritative, for example? With an alter ego, because you're not bound by doubt or fear, you can take on goals you normally wouldn't. Todd Herman, the author of *The Alter Ego Effect*, believes we have two images of ourselves: the one we are right now and the one we dream of being. To inhabit the second one we have to be very clear about how they would act in any given situation, so we can start becoming them. What are their traits? What is their personality like and what are their mindsets? What is their back story? How do you want them to react to different situations? What is your persona's name? What kinds of clothes do they wear?

Like the Romans, emulating role models can be done in many ways. A boxer friend of mine used to channel his long-passed grandfather, who had been a regimental champ, before he climbed in the ring. He did this by eating a Victory V sweet, something his grandfather used to keep in his pocket. If it's a famous historical figure you're channelling, watch them on YouTube, or look at a photo of them. Having a ritual, or a trigger, can help you get into your alter ego role.

What can also help is to write a list of words that describe your alter ego. If you're stuck, think of someone alive or dead that you admire and write down their most admirable traits. Try modifying your daily habits and routines to match your alter ego. If the first alter ego you create doesn't work, design another.

The Importance of Having a Good Role Model – The Greatest

My brothers have all done well because they've got a good work ethic. We all learnt from my dad that if you want something in life then you have to graft for it. He sold carpets door-to-door and moved around a lot. Eventually he got tired of constantly upping sticks and he put down roots in Styal, Cheshire. He was one of the first Travellers in his community to do so, which was seriously going against the grain. Some Travellers said he'd crossed over to the other side with the 'settled folk'. My dad was a maverick and not one to be boxed in. I guess I learnt to be my own man from him.

We all grow up with heroes, and although I don't entertain any these days, Muhammad Ali had a big effect on me, not just as a boxer but also as a man. In my living room in Morecambe I have two very special books. One is a collector's edition book about the Rumble in the Jungle in 1974, published by Taschen and produced with amazing photographs from the fight. The other is a portfolio of very rare photographs of Ali that I was given after I became heavyweight champion of the world. The photos were taken during one of Ali's final photoshoots just before he died in 2016, but he was still smiling. Whenever I look at these photos and the book I am inspired.

What made him so special was that Ali used his celebrity, stepped out of the sporting world, put his head above the parapet and rose to the challenge of standing up for civil rights. He was more than a boxer. When I stepped up and talked about my mental struggles it felt good to do so. In my own small way I felt like I was taking a lesson from the great man himself.

Ali always loved his country but he refused to be drafted into the army in 1967 to fight in Vietnam. 'I ain't got no quarrel with them Vietcong,' he said. He was convicted of draft evasion, sentenced to five years in prison and banned from boxing in the US for three years. It cost him his prime years as a boxer, he lost his livelihood and was stripped of his titles. But through all this he never recanted and remained true to his beliefs. 'I know where I'm going and I know the truth, and I don't have to be what you want me to be. I'm free to be what I want.'

Ali never went into a fight having said good things about his opponent. Every syllable was carefully chosen to weaken them. I've learnt from him in that department! It was always the same message: Ali's opponents were not good enough to cope with his superior skills. Not that he meant a word of the trash talking, it was just the theatre he brought with him, the sheer force of his charisma and character. And yet in the ring there was something of the gentleman about him. He relished the sport, the craft and his God-given ability to dodge ten punches in a row while hemmed in a corner, or the grace with which he could dance across the canvas square. When Ali threw a flurry of punches, the speed and accuracy of his fists was something to behold; it was as if he could even charm time into slowing down. While there are a number of equally skilled boxers, none possessed the charisma and presence that Ali displayed not just in the ring but also in life.

During his career, Ali went from being feted to hated, then loved and admired as an old man suffering from

Parkinson's disease. Towards the end of his life, when asked why, unlike the old days when he was public enemy number one, people now loved him, Ali held up his shaking paw and said: 'It's because I'm more human now. It's the God in people that connects them to me.'

There will never be another Ali. His beauty, skill, compassion, charisma, bravado, sense of play, and, at the end of his life, his humility . . . he truly was the Greatest. If you're looking for a role model to develop your own alter ego, look no further.

Now you're ready for the final round. You've hung in this far, let's smash it!

MOVING FORWARD

FURIOUS WORKOUT XII

One last workout, Team Fury. Let's hear it: WE ARE SPARTANS!

2 Minute Warm-up

- Jog on the spot for 20 sec
- Toe touches x 10
- Cross your legs, slowly touch toes for 10 sec x 2
- Bounce on the spot for 20 sec
- Swivel your hips for 20 sec, then the opposite way for 20 sec
- Kick legs out and shake for 10 sec

30 Minute Session

(Remember: hydrate and rest for 30 sec after each set, x 3 sets)

- Freestyle shadow boxing for 1 minute
- Jump squats x 25
- Press-ups x 15
- Sit-ups x 25
- Bicycle sit-ups x 25
- Half sit-ups/stomach crunches x 25
- Jogging on the spot: left straight punch, right straight punch for 30 sec
- Leg lunges x 25
- Burpees x 25

Warm-down

- Sit on floor, legs straight out, touch toes
- On floor, one leg straight, one leg in, touch toes for 10 sec then switch leg
- On floor, back straight, feet back and pressed together, push thighs down for 10 sec
- Standing up, pull one knee up, holding foot with hand, feel burn in thigh, switch leg
- Rotate hips for 30 sec then switch in other direction

22 February 2020: MGM Grand Garden Arena, Las Vegas, USA

Let's finish where we began this book: Las Vegas. Wilder II. Round Three. Thirty seconds to go. Wilder has beaten the count after I knocked him down.

We lock horns once again in the final seconds of the round. The crowd are on their feet as I drive Wilder against the ropes; his legs are all over the place. He begins to slide down towards the canvas again, as if he's a cartoon character that's just walked into a lamp post. He lurches forward and grabs me for support as if rugby tackling me. I step back and he's on the floor again. It's almost painful to watch. But he's nothing if not strong of heart and determined. That's what I like about Deontay, he's a true gutsy champ and he puts it all on the line. He's either going to win or go out on his shield.

The ref calls it a slip, not a knockdown. Wilder is mercifully saved by the bell. I stare at him as he goes back to his corner. The atmosphere is electric now in the arena; the crowd scent blood. The noise is getting louder and louder. I thrive on it. The Gypsy King thrives on it.

Round Four. We're in Wilder's corner and he's trying hard to remain upright. I'm in the centre of the ring driving him around like a rice farmer with a yoked buffalo. A minute in and he flicks a jab, which I respond to with a jab of my own, followed by a haymaker which he ducks and then he trips on my foot and goes reeling backwards, flying back down to the canvas. I've got plenty of juice left in my tank. I've never felt in finer form. I feel as if there is some divine intervention at work in my fists tonight, the stars are aligning on this historic evening in Vegas. It's one of those rare occasions when things just fall into place.

Still Round Four, unfortunately for Wilder, and I'm gunning him with an orthodox jab until I switch to southpaw and flick a right-hand jab into his face. I spend the rest of the round clinching (holding on to him), wearing him down and offloading heavy rights. If he was a fuel gauge in a car, Wilder would be flashing amber and reading 'empty' by now. He's running on the fumes of instinct. His explosive right hand is now soggy and slow. I feel like I've sapped him of even more energy and strength. Behind a bank of microphones and monitors are the British boxing pundits, among them David Haye, who I later learn was erupting with over-the-top platitudes: 'Tyson Fury is showing how great he is. I don't know of any other heavyweight in the world or in history who could do to Wilder what Fury is doing tonight.'

Round Five and straight away I pepper Wilder with yet more jabs and some big overhead right hands, all of which connect. Wilder stumbles in the corner and clinches for want of something to lean on – and soon regrets it. Bad move, dosser. With the extra weight I'm carrying I'm able to wheel him around to wherever I want him. He feels floppy as a ragdoll in my arms. The fire has been gone from his belly ever since the end of the first round, but now he's markedly groggy, in the throes of defeat, his lip split, his ear a rose of blood. I hit him with a left hook followed by a body shot and he folds upon my fist and down he goes. As are the rules of the game, with my opponent down I trot back to a neutral corner.

All I need is a clear shot now and that's it, game over. But Wilder has the heart of a lion, albeit one on drunken feet. It's in these moments that you reveal your true spirit; you're either a quitter or a fighter, and there's no inch of capitulation in this man. He's facing a living hell where everything is a blur before him; his legs are betraying him as if he's wearing old-fashioned weighted diving boots; he's out of puff and ideas. Perhaps it's muscle memory that ratchets his famous right fist back as if drawing an arrow. He lets it fly towards my head, but it's so clearly telegraphed that I barely have to duck. Wilder stumbles and but for the ropes holding him up he'd be on the canvas again. I work him with heavy right-hand punches and it feels like butchery. While the ref Kenny Bayless has done a great job of keeping the action going, part of me thinks it should be over now. Wilder's taken enough punishment and is in no shape to continue. I lose a point for a late punch and the round finishes in a swarm of yet more stinging shots from the Gypsy King.

When you're dog-tired, when your opponent has taken everything out of you and you're on your last legs, what you fall back on is technical ability, experience and heart. Wilder is nothing but heart. He has no experience of being this ragged, this overwhelmed and outboxed; no experience he can draw on to inspire him to get out of trouble. Unfortunately for him, his technical ability has so many holes in it he's now like a stationary target. But Wilder has never been beaten, and perhaps it is this that fires him up in the sixth round as he comes out from his corner, shoulders twitching. This time it's toe-to-toe streetfighting. It's not the cleanest boxing, and being up close and in my face is not a place the Bronze Bomber feels comfortable. It makes no difference to me. By now he's as weak as a kitten and I'm all but walking through his punches, looking for the knockout as the bell rings at the end of the sixth round. While it may be only half-way through the fight, I sense it won't go the distance, or even another full round. As I sit in my corner, my cut-man unconcerned by the few scuffs on my face, SugarHill, cool as a cucumber, tells me not to get cocky. There's a sense of inevitability in the air; it will all be over soon. But I have to stay focused and concentrate. In victory, stay disciplined.

I jog out for the start of the seventh, feeling sprightly and light on my feet. Wilder looks focused but his body is betraying him, for while he's looking for a window of opportunity to throw his killer right hand, he barely has the energy to lift his 10-ounce gloves. I double-feint him, land a heavy right, then I snap a jab, which rocks his head back. Wilder connects with one good right hand, but for the most part he's swinging wildly. A moment later I have him pinned in the corner and am firing direct jabs like a nail gun; one after the other, they pierce his guard and find their target on his face. Another one-two combination, a body shot and then the crowd erupts as something white flies through the air. In his peripheral vision Kenny Bayless sees the towel land and wades in to stop the barrage of my punches.

I don't remember a great deal else about the fight after this. So much adrenaline was popping through my veins like champagne bubbles, it's hard to describe the euphoria. The crowd was mostly a blur as I was lifted up on my brother Shane and SugarHill's shoulders. I grabbed the mic and thanked Jesus Christ and my team for getting me back. I announced that the king of the heavyweight division had returned. And I launched into a karaoke version of 'American Pie', which the crowd lapped up, singing along to the chorus – even my American promotor Bob Arum, who's in his eighties, belted out a few lines. I hugged Paris and my brothers and team. Team Fury had done it.

And so this particular duel is over, destiny is written and my comeback is complete. I'm not one for looking back, I like to move forward and be in the present, but I think as an old man I may just remember this night. What would the Gypsy Kings of old have made of the performance if they were sitting ringside? 'Job well done, lad,' perhaps.

• • •

You need to be willing to go the distance in life. Sometimes, like during my Wilder II fight, you'll be pleasantly surprised and find that the moment when you take on your greatest challenge won't be the war of attrition you had planned for. But being ready for a drawn-out battle is the only way I believe that you can have the confidence and the belief to achieve a win of any kind.

In this last round, rather than fixate on the final bell that rings to say your challenge is over, I want us to take one final look at being present and in the moment, how to enjoy the 'now' and take pleasure from life's journey, and how to move forward. Moving forward was the boxing strategy I used in the ring to beat Wilder; I wasn't afraid to take the fight to him. But moving forward in life in general is something we all have to encounter after we've attempted a goal. And although it may sound counter-intuitive, and regardless of whether you achieve your goal or not, it's a mindset rooted in the present that will guide you towards your next challenges in life. Without this presence of mind, you can feel a bit lost after you've completed a big task and, like me after my victory against Wladimir Klitschko, can be left asking yourself what's left to do.

Recently, I went back to my old gym in Lancaster where I first danced under the lights as a lad. Nothing much had changed; there are still exposed brick walls, taped-up heavy bags and the smell of dirty wraps, leather gloves and sweat all mixed together. Sometimes you have to go back to where your journey began to realise how far you've come. Back then it was all a dream and a vision, and now that dream and vision have become a reality. As I stood there with the ghost of my younger self firing out jabs in a mirror, watched over by a poster of Jesus pasted to the wall, I thought to myself, what a strange and wonderful thing life is. Rather than being merely nostalgic, this kind of thinking is important, as it helped me celebrate my success even more. If we don't celebrate our successes, if we move on too quickly, it can leave us in a funk.

Life is good for me at the minute. I'm training regularly, eating clean, and I have my family around me.

I've nothing to be down about. When I'm older I'm sure I'll be able to look back on this time and remember it as a golden period: I'm fit and healthy, my wife and I are in our prime, our kids are happy and I still have my mum and dad. I live for today, having spent many years waiting to have this feeling, thinking what I would do when I was world champ. I never lived in the moment before as I was always thinking about winning and beating the next opponent. But now that I've got here, I love what I've achieved. I set my targets for what I was going to do, and I delivered on them. I wasn't a finisher with other things in life, even with small things like books and video games. But boxing was different, it was my destiny.

They say you get to know the real 'you' through experiencing adversity. I'm thankful for the journey I've been on as my eyes have now been opened to the things that really matter and the things that don't. People who glide through life without getting to the deep or choppy water only see the surface of things and lack the depth of someone who has sunk to the bottom and fought hard to swim back up to the light. It's only then that you can truly appreciate how precious a thing this life is. Like the boxing scars I have on my face, I'm proud of my mental scars, too. And you should be proud of yours.

I'm grateful for the now, and that the future is something to look forward to rather than something I dread. You can't live your life for tomorrow, telling yourself things will be better when you've got this or done that. They won't be better unless you make it happen now. It's a cliché, but life is really not just about the destination, it's about the journey too, and learning to enjoy the twists and turns en route to the final bell in Round Twelve.

So, practically speaking, how do you immerse yourself in the now? There are lots of different approaches. It's important to listen to our family and friends. Look people in the eye and be curious about their journey and their story. An approach that many people take to live for today is to take time to stop and smell the air, to enjoy the weather and the change of the seasons, to notice things gradually turning. We're all going in only one direction, so let's enjoy it, and not waste time lost in worry. It's not worth it. There are so many things that you can do. Below are some of the most popular things people reflect upon on their deathbeds, which I think are a good steer to help us live better now:

- **I wish I'd stopped over-thinking things and just gone for it**
  Ask yourself how many exciting things you talk yourself out of because they are out of your comfort zone and represent change and uncertainty.
  Remember: change only comes when there is a

vacuum that must be filled, i.e., when you have taken the old away, making room for the new.

- **I wish I hadn't settled for a job I didn't like**
As Jim Carrey said: 'You can fail at what you don't want, so you might as well take a chance doing what you love.' Who is to say you can't be anything you want to evolve into? The restrictions we apply to ourselves are glass ceilings that need to be smashed. When you give yourself permission to chase your calling, passion or dream, your mind and body get in flow with each other and this is when the magic happens; it suddenly becomes natural and easy to achieve what you want. Could you expect that from a job where you just turn up for the money?

- **I wish I hadn't worried so much about what other people thought of me**
In *Game of Thrones*, George R.R. Martin had one of his characters discuss the idea that a lion never gets advice from sheep. It's true. Don't be a herd member if you want to do great things. Be your own person, have the strength to stand by your own opinions, and have the confidence to believe your ideas are good enough to be successful. Believe me, most people are dealing with their

own problems in life and haven't got time to think about you as much as you might think.

- **I wish I had taken more risks**
  Those who play it safe throughout their life look back and wish they had injected a bit more colour and strayed from the well-trodden path to take a chance on something that might have failed but might also have triumphed. Those who take risks see more of the world and more of their own inner landscape; they travel in themselves and learn much more about themselves.

- **I wish I'd dedicated myself to growing some of my dreams into reality**
  All of us are capable of dreaming, but not so many of us are willing to tend to our secret goal and guide and nurture it over a long period of time. You reap what you sow.

- **I wish I hadn't given up on my goal at the first hurdle**
  Sometimes it can seem as if we don't want to actually achieve our goals, because then we can go back to the safety of the familiar and say, 'Well, at least I tried.' It is those who dust themselves off

after a fall, or having been knocked down get
straight back up, who succeed.

- **I wish I'd told others how much I loved them**
  We all know that nobody is around for ever, so why
  wait till those you love are gone before you tell them
  how special they are to you? Think of someone right
  now who means a lot to you. Call them.

- **I wish I'd taken better care of my body**
  Your body is a reflection of what you do with it day
  to day, and how highly you regard yourself. If you
  have more respect for your body, you'll have more
  respect for yourself. You don't have to live like a
  monk; moderation is the key. If I want some
  chocolate, I buy some. But you don't want a body
  that chocolate built. Take care of your body and
  you'll feel better.

- **I wish I'd not held on to old grudges**
  As I've said before in this book, giving into a grudge
  is like holding a burning coal in your palm. You're
  the one who gets hurt, while the other person is
  often oblivious. It's wasted energy and it's toxic, so
  move on; forgive and forget. If that's not possible,
  air your grievance with them and try to start afresh.

- **I wish I'd stayed in touch with friends**
  Good friends are worth their weight in gold
  and essential for fighting off loneliness and
  depression. A trusted old friend is someone who
  knows you like no other and forgives you your
  weaknesses. Don't be the stubborn one who waits
  for them to call. Pick up the phone and connect.

- **I wish I had trusted my instincts**
  The more we get to know ourselves, the more
  familiar we are with that inner voice inside our heads,
  which actually often isn't in our head but in our gut.
  Apparently, the human stomach has more neurons
  than a cat's brain. That's why gut feelings are so
  strong. There's a reason we have them: when we were
  lower in the food chain they kept us alive. These days
  we get intuitive gut feelings about people and more
  often than not they are proved to be correct.

How many of these lessons will you apply to the rest of
your days? All of them? Half of them? The only way to make
sure you don't end up filled with regrets is to make a change
right now. If you didn't fill in the goal section in Round
Three, then please go back to it now. Before you write
anything, take some time, make a cup of tea, put your
feet up and let your mind wander. Don't be thinking about

your gas bill, the fact you're almost out of milk, or you haven't hoovered today. Relax, breathe deeply and allow your mind to focus on where you hoped you would be at this time of your life. What would you still like to do?

One of the learnings from the list above is: don't live your life for other people, live it for yourself. It's so important to carve out time for yourself and your partner. My wife Paris is my rock and my best friend. She's ringside at every fight, even though she hates watching me fight. She ducks and dodges in her seat as if it is her in the ring and absorbs every punch that gets through to me. She's my talisman and my true North. We've been together since our teens but we still make time for one another on dates. A relationship doesn't keep moving on its own; it needs care and love.

On that point, I don't think you experience pure love until you have kids. These little versions of yourself are a part of you, they came from you and have your blood flowing through their veins. The love I get from my kids is the best thing in my life. To love and be loved – nothing comes close to it. If we go broke and have to eat stale cheese sandwiches, so be it. If we have each other we have everything. If I lived in a cardboard box with my family, we'd still be happy because we're all in it together. If one goes down, we all go down together. As long as they are in my life and they love me, nothing else matters.

My five kids drive me bonkers at times but I love them more than life itself. Not so long ago I thought the best view in the world was out of a Vegas penthouse, but these days my favourite thing is the sight of my kids wandering into the bedroom first thing in the morning and waking me up with a sleepy smile, or when one of the little ones wants a bottle making up. I love doing things for them: getting their breakfast ready in the week, taking them to school and picking them up. It's hard to describe the love you feel for your kids. My oldest two have come to watch me box only the once and it was a bit much for them. It's better if they watch it on TV because then at least it can be paused if things are going south. Will my kids follow in their dad's footsteps? Who can say? Certainly, it's in their DNA. But the real point of saying all of this is that I'm living in the present, for the first time in a long time. And I'm so much happier for it.

. . .

A Furious Future

When I think of the future, I'm none the wiser as to when I'll hang up my gloves for good. Time doesn't stand still for anyone, especially boxers, so it won't be long. There's a short story called 'A Piece of Steak' by the writer Jack London that someone told me about. In it, Tom King, a journeyman boxer with his best fighting years long behind him, has to fight Sandel, a young up-and-coming boxer. The problem is that Tom can't afford to eat before the fight; if he had a steak in his stomach he might just have the fuel to win. He knows his only chance against the young fighter is to use his experience, and as the fight begins Tom throws all his tricks at his opponent because he knows his body won't last the distance, tired as it is with age and a lack of fuel. He puts Sandel down on the canvas and he seems out for the count but 'youth' rallies inside the younger boxer and he quickly recovers, picks himself up and wins the fight. The message is clear: the old must always make way for the young to come through.

You can't beat time and youth is as irrepressible as the incoming tide in Morecambe Bay beyond my open window. There is no point in me waiting for the likes of Daniel Dubois to come of age as a fighter. I've done everything and more that I set out to do in the sport. I reckon I've got another two or three fights left and then I'll retire and focus my efforts on helping young people find their way through sport and continue to fly the flag for mental health. Once I've retired, that's it. You won't see me making a comeback, though it seems to be very popular at the minute with the likes of Oscar De La

Hoya, Mike Tyson and Roy Jones Jr dusting off their gloves to return to the ring! Is it because the tiger misses the hunt, or do they just need to make some money? Just because you get older it doesn't mean your love of the fight game fades. Your body may weaken but the fire that burns in all former champion boxers never goes out.

And fair play to them, so long as they don't get hurt. George Foreman was world champ at forty-five, and Bernard Hopkins became a world champ again at forty-six years of age. Archie Moore, Foreman's coach, fought professionally until he was forty-seven. Floyd Mayweather too often talks about coming back. Fighters like him feed off the fight game. Without it, perhaps he's just a normal 10 stone, 5 foot 7 guy who blends into the background. For all his money, private jets and his extraordinary boxing talent and achievement, if you saw Mayweather in a restaurant without his entourage of bodyguards, and a fleet of Bugatti Veyrons and Rolls-Royce Phantoms lined up outside, you might not notice anything special about him. But, ultimately, my advice to anyone on knowing when the time is right to retire is that it's down to you. Go out on your terms. Who am I to judge?

Whenever I decide to hang up my gloves, at least I know what I want to do next, because along my journey I've realised that I get more joy out of helping other people than I do in helping myself. There's a reason volunteers are happy to offer their time and get paid nothing for it: the feeling that lights their insides after they've helped someone is something money can't buy. When we do things for others it feels natural, as if this is something we were designed to do. Not surprisingly it has been proved to help fight depression and lower blood pressure, as well as build social connections, which in turn helps combat loneliness.

In an interview after the first Wilder fight I revealed my mental-health demons to the world. I hadn't prepared the words, I never do, but I've never been so clear on anything: 'I showed the world tonight, and everyone suffering with mental-health problems, you can come back and it can be done. Everyone out there who has the same problems I've been suffering with, I did that for you guys. And if I can come back from where I came from then you can do it too. So get up, get over it, seek help and let's do it as a team.'

I knew this speech was going out to millions of homes around the world and would be viewed by people suffering in silence with depression because of the stigma attached to the illness. It was the beginning of a change in me; I was becoming less interested in myself and more concerned with the plight of others. It was time for me to start giving something back. Since then I've become known for speaking out about mental health and it's not unusual for me to get the odd visit from someone who is struggling – even in the middle of the night. I was a bit freaked out but also humbled when, in December 2019, a lad in his twenties knocked on our door. It was still way before dawn. He told me he was having suicidal thoughts and he needed to speak to me before he did anything. I took him out on a three-mile run and we talked about what he was going through and how he was feeling. Thankfully he felt better for it and I recommended he get professional help immediately.* He left in a much better mood, and I think he began the long journey of confronting and managing his depression. Only the other day I

---

* Just to say again, I'm not an expert. If you're experiencing suicidal thoughts, or you know someone who is, I urge you to get professional help immediately. There are great free helplines, such as the Samaritans, who are on-hand right now to support you and guide you through this difficult time. You can also talk to someone you trust – family or friends. You're not on your own. As the NHS say on their website, 'there's no right or wrong way to talk about suicidal feelings – starting the conversation is what's important.' You can also contact your GP or call the NHS on 111. If you or someone you know is in danger, contact emergency services or seek medical aid immediately. At the back of this book you'll find a list of mental-health resources, that may be of help. Call or email them if you need help, but do it *now*. It's the little first steps we take that are the greatest on our journey.

bumped into him on the beach and he seemed a lot better in himself. If I can help people experiencing difficulty in their lives as a result of mental-health issues, it's something I'm enormously proud to do.

Since I started putting my thoughts into words in this book, Vinnie Jones has spoken out about his own struggles. When he tells people he has depression they look at him like he's an axe murderer; he then feels compelled to add that it's because he's grieving over his wife's death. We need more people like Vinnie taking a risk to talk about their dark times and to share their struggles if we're to really remove the stigma of depression. We can all open up more with each other. I urge you to do so too.

I believe we should all aim to help those in our communities who are less fortunate than ourselves, in any ways we can. Arnold Schwarzenegger once said: 'You can only feel complete as a person when you think about how you can help your fellow members [of the human race].' I now know my future is about putting myself in the service of others who need a break in life, like the homeless. We need to remember that it could so easily be us sitting scared and vulnerable in a doorway, shivering in a sleeping bag. They weren't born homeless. Often, something happened that sent them on a downward spiral: their loved ones died, they lost their job, they were abused, or fell prey to addiction to numb the pain of their trauma. They're humans, not someone we should pretend isn't there as we walk by.

I also want to inspire young people. I recently set up the Tyson Fury Foundation to help promote outdoor activity among young people and give kids from poor backgrounds the chance to shine through sport. One way the foundation will work is through a new gym in Morecambe that we've bought. Close to the football club, it has four and a half acres of land that will be used for football pitches, basketball, netball and rugby. Unlike the boxing gyms of my youth, the equipment is all state-of-the-art and new.

I've asked my good pal Shaun to be the ambassador for the foundation. He has so much experience working with people who have difficulties, whether it's helping recently paralysed individuals get used to their wheelchairs or empowering young people with special needs to get involved in sport. Shaun is working on becoming the first qualified disabled divemaster, which sends a very clear message out to all those people who have special needs that extraordinary things can be achieved, and that the treasures of the deep are open to all. Shaun set up the Lancaster Bulldogs, a wheelchair basketball club for people with all kinds of disabilities. He tells them that nothing is impossible. I've popped down to watch them train and they inspire me so much. I remember one of the juniors was a sweet girl with cerebral palsy who I learnt was being bullied online. Shaun asked me to talk to her and I put a picture of us on my Instagram site, which went viral. Apparently, she got more respect as a result of that photo and the bullying stopped. Up until this point I hadn't realised what a positive impact I could have on young people.

As a kid I lived outside. We played hide and seek in the woods, made games up, rode our bikes or ripped about the fields on motorbikes. Outside was for playing. Inside was a place you went when it was dark or raining and it was boring. I think kids these days spend far too much time inside, glued to their PlayStations and Xboxes, slaves to their phones, laptops and iPads. Think how large a chunk of our kids' lives is being swallowed up doing the same thing day after day. I recently banned my kids from being on their phones and iPads because they were getting obsessed and becoming unsociable. It's funny how quickly they come back to normal when their attention is not taken up by a gadget. I hope that, even in a small way, my foundation can help get kids active and outside.

After Wilder II, Lancaster and Morecambe council asked me if I would like a statue of myself erected, or have a victory parade through the streets to celebrate my new WBC world title. I told them I wasn't interested in anything like that. But putting something back into the place where I live and giving young people an opportunity to do something positive with their lives and try new sports, that excites me. As I've said in this book, sport develops our bodies, builds character through working as part of a team, and makes us push through pain and fatigue. It helps us to find resolve in difficult times and teaches us to learn to handle losing with dignity; losing is just a part of life. As well as helping kids at a grassroots level find their way in sport, the Tyson Fury Foundation is going to help educate young offenders who have just come out of jail and help them stay on the straight and narrow. If I manage all of that, I also want to bring training camps to Morecambe one day, to create a space where boxers will come to prepare for big fights. It makes me feel good, knowing that I can make a difference. And although I'm now in a privileged position and we might not all be able to set up our own foundation, we can all do our bit to help others less well-off than ourselves.

A few nights ago, me and my dad were training on the beach in Morecambe on the boxing pads. We'd made an announcement on social media that we'd be doing it and given people two hours to get there if they wanted to see me training. It was a warm evening beneath a clear sky and it felt great getting lots of people of all ages outdoors. Some people focus their charity on overseas problems, but I'd rather contribute to my local area. Bin men, policemen, firemen, NHS workers; they are all unsung heroes. Throughout the pandemic, and beyond, they continue to keep us going. They do a fantastic job and are not recognised enough.

* * *

It's been a pleasure writing this book for you. My hope is that I might have been able to inspire some of you out there battling poor mental health to seek advice from those who can really help you, as I did, and to find sanctuary and sanity through the power of daily exercise. Equally, for those readers looking to find direction in their lives, or to turn pipe dreams into tangible goals and move forward towards achieving them, I hope you will have found a few useful nuggets of wisdom here.

Up North, we have the most dramatic skies. Where I live in particular, the light changes from one moment to the next, from black storm clouds over the Irish Sea, to hopeful sunshine lighting the white sands of the beach. Not so different to our moods then. We can all go from sad to happy in the blink of an eye. So remember this: when you're down, there will always be light on the way and the sooner you force a smile in the dark and gather your gratitude around you, the quicker you'll find your way back to the sunshine. By embracing your courage and living each day as your last, I pray that none of you ever loses hope in life or in yourself. I believe in you.

Below are twelve final tips from me to live a happier and more fulfilled life, summing up the things we've looked at in this book. Thanks for your company, mush. It's been fun. Now, if you don't mind, it's time for me to go training. You coming?

Twelve Ways to Live a Happier & More Furious Life

Exercise every day: This is the single most important factor for me in managing my mental health. Don't kid yourself you don't need it. Exercise keeps your heart pumping blood around your body and it keeps you young.

Eat healthily: By learning a bit more about the food we eat we can make choices about how much energy we have and how healthy we feel. We are what we eat. Hydrating regularly keeps the gut clean too.

Avoid watching the news: I feel like the news is almost designed to scare us sometimes. It can be negative and alarmist. Turn it off if it's getting you down.

Face your fears: Maybe your version of Deontay Wilder is a credit card bill that needs to be dealt with, or a relationship that needs to be finished. Whatever it is that keeps you awake at night, the sooner you're free of it, the sooner you'll give yourself some mental peace.

Practise gratitude: Life is what you make of it. Focus on being grateful for the good things. If you tell yourself you are lucky it emits a kind of beacon in the darkness and other good things come towards your light. We get what we attract.

Don't live on social media: It can be a waste of time. A lot of the content on it is rubbish. Some people are more interested in following other people's lives than getting on with their own. Live your own life, not someone else's.

Don't let your kids grow up too soon – and don't forget to be a kid: Kids want to grow up and be adults straight away, while adults look back to their youth and wistfully wish they were young again. The grass is always greener on the other side of the fence. Be a child as long as you can because before you know it you will be burdened with responsibility, and there's plenty of time for that. And if you are an adult, don't forget to allow yourself to be a kid sometimes. Nobody is marking you down for having fun and laughing.

Go best or go home: Don't do second or third place in life. My aim was always to be number one. Set your stall out very high so even if you don't quite get where you wanted to go, you'll still get somewhere good. If you aim for the stars and get to the moon you've done well.

Get plenty of sleep: You need to go to bed at the same time each night and get plenty of rest for your mind and body to recuperate from the efforts of the day.

Focus on what you are doing: Keep your head down. Life is not a race against your fellow human beings; it's a race against time. That's your only concern, that you are not filling your days to their optimum.

Don't focus on everyone else around you: Stop looking at how well this person or that person is doing, or how much better someone might be at doing something than you. Everyone has different skillsets. If you are determined and practised, you too will become an expert in your chosen field.

Enjoy the now: When it comes to time, you either use it or you lose it. Life is too short for regrets. What we did yesterday is history. It's about living for today, savouring the moment and being thankful for what we have in the present, not what we think we want in the future.

MENTAL HEALTH CONTACTS & HELPLINES

As I mentioned at the start of this book, if you have been affected by mental health problems and have experienced or are experiencing suicidal thoughts, please get professional medical help immediately – contact the NHS on 111, or speak to a doctor or your GP. If you or someone you know is in danger, please contact emergency services immediately. Below is a list of mental health resources for you to explore, alongside seeking professional help.

Mind

mind.org.uk

Mind is one of the best-known UK charities devoted to helping people with mental health problems. It has around 125 local offices in England and Wales, which offer services including talking therapies, peer support, crisis care and housing support. In order to find the closest Mind to you go to: mind.org.uk/information-support/local-minds/

Anxiety Care UK

anxietycare.org.uk

Anxiety UK

03444 775774 (Monday – Friday, 9.30am – 5.30pm)
anxietyuk.org.uk

Advice and support for people living with anxiety, stress, anxiety-based depression or phobias.

British Association for Counselling and Psychotherapy (BACP)

01455 883300
bacp.co.uk

Provides information about counselling and therapy, and has a directory so you can find a therapist near you.

Improving Access to Psychological Therapies (IAPT)

nhs.uk/service-search

Use the NHS search page to find psychological therapies services near you.

The National Institute for Health and Care Excellence (NICE)

nice.org.uk

Information and clinical guidelines on recommended treatments for different conditions, including anxiety disorders.

No More Panic

nomorepanic.co.uk

Provides information, support and advice for those with panic disorder, anxiety, phobias and OCD, including a forum and chat room.

No Panic

0844 967 4848 (daily, 10am – 10pm)
nopanic.org.uk

Provides a helpline, step-by-step programmes, and support for those with anxiety disorders.

Samaritans

116 123 (24-hour service)

samaritans.org

Emotional support for anyone who needs to talk. Calls are free from all providers and do not appear on bills.

Triumph Over Phobia (TOP UK)

topuk.org

Provides self-help therapy groups and support for those with OCD, phobias and related anxiety disorders.

The Frank Bruno Foundation

thefrankbrunofoundation.co.uk

The Frank Bruno Foundation provides support, encouragement and the motivation to succeed for those facing and recovering from mental ill health.

INDEX

Page references in *italics* indicate images.

TF indicates Tyson Fury.